You don't have to be Superman to be a Superdad

9 traits of a Superdad

Adam Schwaegerman

You don't have to be Superman to be a Superdad

9 Traits of a Superdad

Adam Schwaegerman

Table of Contents

Dedication

This book is dedicated to the three people on this planet that know me best, my good and my bad, and choose to love me regardless. They accept me for what I am, what I am not, and love me unconditionally. I can never fully convey how much you all mean to me.

Fran, you have been my rock and my north star. When dark days hit, you're always there. You never waver in your love for me. When I fall short, you never waver in your love for me. You are such a picture of God's love. Without you my life would have no flavor or taste. You make me want to be a better man each day.

Jayden, you are the best person I know. You've helped me more than you know. I am sober today because of your courage and support. You are best buddy, my inspiration, and son. You inspire me to be a better man each day.

Bella, you are my sweet angel. You remind me so much of my mother with your loving kindness towards others, even strangers. I cannot imagine the countless ways you will make an impact on this world. You have such a sweet spirit that makes me want to be a better man each day.

Introduction

"Continuous improvement is better than delayed perfection"

-Mark Twain

I have made more mistakes than any parent I know. I set out my day with a morning meditation centered around patience and then lose patience with my wife, bark at my daughter, and snap at my son. I've failed again and again at being a perfect dad. So why write a book on parenting, you ask?

Great question! I am writing down what I wish my younger self knew. I am sharing my lessons forged through my fire of failure so future dads, like my son and students, won't have to repeat the same mistakes. You see, I refuse to quit trying to be a Superdad because I believe these traits can be learned and internalized.

Why do most self-help and parenting books ultimately fail and fall short of delivering their promised result? We start something, only to see if disappear in a week, month, year. Is it because we don't have a good plan? Perhaps we just weren't disciplined enough? There are probably enough answers to that question to fill this book and many more.

Before we start looking traits of a Superdad, we must recognize that we are human. No matter how hard we work at something we will always makes mistakes. There is no such thing as a perfect dad. For that matter, our kids are imperfect too. We will screw up, overreact when the kids mess up and generally blow it. It is a factor of the human condition. It is also what makes life interesting.

Can you imagine we're all perfect with no complications, like some kind of simulation? Sound good? There would be no recovery, no triumph, no forgiveness, no redemption. We must accept that life is messy. A beautiful mess if you will. There is no one perfect way to parent. Each parent is different, and each child is different. This book does not attempt to create yet another artificial standard for parents to beat themselves up over. We do that enough already!

Rather, we wanted to put together a compilation of the traits we should all strive for, fathers *and* mothers. Vince Lombardi once said,

"Perfection is not attainable, but if we chase perfection, we can attain excellence." While perfection is an unattainable goal, we all want to be better parents. We believe these traits to be the foundation of great parents. We may not be perfect dads, but we can be Superdads.

We've put this book together as a meditation for parents, rather than a list. Besides, when is the last time a list worked for you? After all, it's *who you are*, not *what you do* that impacts your children's lives. This book provides practical suggestions to improve your relationship with your children. We're talking about assimilation here, not simply acting. Internalization is the difficult work of parenting, but it is so beautiful.

I am writing this book as a collection of traits for other dads like me, who didn't have a great example to follow. Truth is, I've made just about every mistake a young father can make. My upbringing did not offer a positive blueprint in raising my children. It has been a trial-and-error approach since day one. This book is not exclusive, nor does it claim these are the only traits of a Superdad. We are all a mosaic, trying to do the best we can with the hand were dealt.

As a product of every form of abuse under the Sun, I learned terribly destructive behavior patterns. Many of these persisted into my early adult years and hung around even after becoming a father. I came to a point in my life where I had two choices: 1) continue to be a victim by blaming my abusive upbringing for my parental failures and immaturity or 2) quit making excuses, humble myself, and accept direction from any and every situation and relationship.

When your children see you admit to your weaknesses, accept help, and then actually try to change, beautiful things happen in your relationships! This humility tears down walls of anger and unforgiveness. It is then that life becomes brighter and sweeter. Now I am not promising roses and butterflies here. But what I am saying is simple, successful parental relationships center around certain traits, and these traits can be learned. You can become a Superdad.

We can become better parents. Are we to stop growing once were "grown"? No way. We must continuously model lifelong learning and growth for our children. They don't do what we say, they do what we do. We set an example for them to follow and repeat. We fathers are here to break every curse and set our children up for success in life. It is our calling to end the generational bondage that we've been passed from hindering our children. Armed with this knowledge, will you join me as we look at the nine traits of a Superdad?

Chapter 1 – Selfless

"The one thing about being a parent is the ability to be selfless: To give up the things you want and need for the benefit of someone else"

-Danny McBride

What attracts you to certain leaders and not others? Who really has your trust? The answer to both of those questions can generally point you towards the qualities of great leadership. Think about a coach, a colleague, a friend, and/or family member that inspires you like no other. Those individuals probably possess an ability to see what is best for you, instead of always looking out for themselves. They can be called selfless because although they recognize their own wants and desires, they can put those aside for the betterment of another. True selflessness is the beginning of love.

Think about it. Do you value a relationship that is a one-way street? Do you surround yourself with people that always seem to ignore your needs while pursuing their wants? We are selfish creatures. We do look out for and constantly pursue selfish desires. But when the universe sends us a person that has the maturity and ability to put aside their selfish desires to advance a greater cause, we stand in awe and want to be near such a person. We want to be friends with someone like that. We will listen to their advice because they have built our trust through proven selflessness. They proved they care about our well-being above their personal agenda.

This trait of selfless love completely contradicts our American economic system. Our entire economy is based on one simple principle, profit motive. What motivates us to wake up and go to work in the morning, profit motive. What motivates companies to produce and sell products, profit motive. We walk up and go to work each day to make a profit. That is a noble cause, to work and pay for one's expenses.

Problem is personal selfishness can and will destroy relationships. Finding the ability to set aside personal wants is the beginning of being a Superdad because without showing your children they're a priority, how can you really lead them? Will they want to follow you once they aren't dependent on you for food, shelter, and necessities? When we prioritize things above our children, we damage the relationship and risk losing our closeness and influence in their lives.

Does this mean all parents must abandon their schedules and priorities? Absolutely not. In my previous book, "My Journey to Heal the Body" I discuss setting priorities and making your health a priority over family obligations. This may sound conflicting and is in no way meant to confuse the principle of selflessness. To be clear, setting exercise and healthy eating priorities is NOT automatically selfish. If your goal is to be healthy, alive, present, and not a burden, then how can that be considered selfish? In fact, it is the opposite. You're making certain that, as far as it depends on you, your health will never be your children's problem. Now if your goals are vain, that can be selfish. The bottom line here is what are you giving up?

Many middle-aged parents lose their health priorities in the busyness of raising children, school events, practices, games, cooking meals, and life in general. We begin to eat unhealthy foods, stop exercising, and portray a bad example for our children. My point is not to make parents feel bad for prioritizing their children. But being selfless does not, and never has equated to never doing nothing for yourself. We are not promoting martyrdom or monastery practices here. We are simply sending the message to our children that they are a priority in our lives through our decisions.

Setting healthy living goals like eating healthy foods and exercising thirty minutes per day are extremely positive examples for our children to follow. Waking up early or setting aside half of a lunch break are excellent strategies to curb the time loss it requires to practice healthy living. If you are missing your children's events to live a healthy life, you are communicating to your children through your actions that you are more important to you than they are. You are sending the message they aren't as important as your personal goals. Consider what you are trading to accomplish your goals. Are you spending hours in the gym to reach your goals but only spending five minutes with your child each day? If so, message sent. And you child notices, whether they tell you or not.

I have a friend who works out more than anyone I've ever known. There is probably someone living in a mountain somewhere in

Montana that has him beat, but not by much. His commitment to physical training and exercise is unparalleled. Over the last twenty years he has modeled healthy exercise habits consistently, rarely missing days, even when pain or sickness arrive. In fact, he is the best shape of his life at the age of 48 and is only getting better.

As we've aged, I always privately wondered how he would balance his health priorities with raising his four children. Things became even more interesting when his children became involved in club and varsity athletics. As parents, we know how difficult it can be with multiple children in multiple activities. Although this friend rarely misses a workout, he *never* misses a game, recital, match, or important event in his children's life. He reminds me through his actions that it can be done. We have time for what really matters to us.

Perhaps you're putting in extra hours at work with the hope of a promotion so you can really prioritize your family. If I can just get to this position, then I can focus on them and make them a priority. How deceptive deception is! That new position will bring more pay and prestige, and with it, more responsibilities. You're plan to be free to focus on your family will only produce frustration and make spending time with them more difficult. Trust me.

How do I know? Because I was that guy! I was a rising star teacher and coach when I married my wife in 2006. I was accustomed to working 14-hour days regularly during basketball season. Sometimes even as much as 18 hours when duty called. When my wife became pregnant with our son in 2007, I dreamed of a day when I could work less, make more, and prioritize my new family. This would be an opportunity to do it right after all the mistakes I watched and suffered as a child.

A new principal took note of my can-do attitude and promoted me to the position of assistant principal after just one year at the age of 30. Of course, this meant I had to go back to school to earn a master's degree and get credentialed as a principal in the state of Texas. Although I was on the fast track, my master's course work kept me in evening and break classes for almost two years. I remember feeling relieved at my graduation because now I could finally go home after school and be with my family.

My new principal had other plans and decided to utilize his newly accredited assistant in committees, administrative meetings, pep rallies, class trips, class meetings, staff meetings, teacher trainings, master schedule collaborations, and many other initiatives. More money = more responsibility. I was even busier than before. Coaching seemed so simple at that point. Now I was managing the students *and* the teachers.

To make matters worse, I felt deserving to attend regular Friday happy hours with other district leadership where I would meet and greet with people who could help advance my career goals. I'm embarrassed to say that I routinely attended these gatherings, while my wife was home with our new son. I genuinely convinced myself that by attending these fraternal gatherings I was ultimately doing it to be with my family. Again, how deceptive deception can be!

Two years passed and I followed my boss to a new district with the promise of more money and time with my family. There I would assume the title "lead assistant principal," which I would learn meant I now managed students, teachers, *and* the other leadership while he was away teaching college classes three days per week. What looked promising quickly turned into not seeing my family awake for days and eventually entire weeks. How did it get to this point? How did I go from a career that was demanding in season to a career that is demanding all the time?

Within months of accepting my new position my grandmother passed away. Just seven weeks later, my mother passed away. I was devasted and depressed. I felt like I was in a bad dream where everyone else was living life and I was stuck grieving in a job that I hated. Faculty there were so kind and warm. But nothing could change my internal voice telling me this wasn't for me. I knew then that I could not be a great husband and father *and* great principal. I would have to make a choice: career or family.

Perhaps some will disagree with that thought, and that is alright. There is enough room at the table for more than one opinion here. I had some of my best friends tell me I was wrong in my assessment, and I was just suffering from "buyers' remorse." However, I can only tell my reality and that was my choice to make. You may know others who balance both and are amazing leaders, spouses, and parents. We have yet to meet one. Most of the parents we know eventually come to a fork in the road and must chose. A career on the fast track that includes night, weekends, and travel or a stable, calmer existence where you can prioritize family.

Fran and I discussed returning to teaching. We discussed the negative impact this would have on my salary. At the time we were a single income family because my wife wasn't a citizen and therefore not legally allowed to work. Could I provide for my new family of four on a teacher's salary? Would we go into debt and lose the house if I make this move? I'll never forget the response my wife had when we pondered these and other questions. "Do what makes you happy. We'll have each other." It was at that moment I knew two things: 1) I married the right woman! And 2) the decision had been made…I'd be a teacher as soon as possible. What an amazing woman!

I informed the boss of my decision to return to the classroom shortly after burying my grandmother and mother but stayed on in my position for an additional year out of loyalty to him. I shared with my new boss that the losses and the news of a second child on the way changed the way I saw my future. I could no longer continue in leadership, and the school deserved someone more dedicated. He completely understood and respected my decision but asked that I stay on while he searched for a replacement.

After an additional year, I returned to teaching and endured a $25,000 pay cut. We were amid a home remodel which I was still paying off, just had our second child, and were clipping coupons to get by. But we were happy. Really happy! I cannot tell you the weight that fell off my shoulder's when I stopped competing to be on top and work for the extras. It is so freeing to just embrace contentment. We had each other. The bills were paid. Our new family was all that mattered.

My new schedule meant I never miss family dinners, basketball practices, games, dance recitals. We were even able to schedule a Tuesday night family gathering with my stepdad so the kids can grow up around him, something we do to this day. Twelve years have passed since that decision, and I'm pleased to say that I'm happier today than the day it was made. My wife is now a U.S. Citizen and happily employed. Even my salary increased beyond what I made in leadership. But what really matters is the time. I have been present at the most important moments of my children's lives. There hasn't been one second where I regretted that decision.

We have one thing in common with Bill Gates, Elon Musk, and Jeff Bezos: We all have 24 hours in a day. What we do with them is up to us. Priorities determine where we invest our time. If we do not set our priorities, we slip into a pattern of wastefulness that is hard to break. Time seems to increase its speed exponentially. In this sense, there is no time to waste. Prioritize your children's lives and events. If it is important to them, it should be to you as well.

You will never regret being present, but you will regret missing their formative years. Do you really want to meet your adult children for dinner and have no context to the person they've become? How had they got there? Yes, you know the result, but know nothing of the struggles, the day-to-day stuff. That is the important stuff in life. I promise you when were on our death beds we won't be worried about a meeting, a workout, a deal, a profit margin. What will matter is **who** is in that room?

Don't wait to be on the table to make them a priority. Do it now. How do start, you ask? I have all these responsibilities and can't just leave them? We're not saying you must make an abrupt turn and abandon your career or company on a whim. Start small. Delegate small meetings, tasks, and trips to free up the time to be present at something. Ask your children what they want you to attend and keep your promise to be present.

Understand the seasons of life. In your career field, there may be busier times than others. You may also experience down times during the year. Target these times to make the investment of spending time with your children. Keep in mind when your busiest times are and try to mitigate that by communicating with them.

As a teacher I enjoy almost a mirrored schedule as my children. This is one of the major factors in my decision to return to the classroom. You see as an administrator you're contract requires an additional six weeks of duty. While my teacher friends were already posting family vacation pictures, I was stuck in meetings. My children were left home, bored. Sure, the extra money provided a few extras when we finally did go on vacation, but in heart I knew I was missing out on the good stuff.

Perhaps leaving your professional isn't realistic and downsizing career goals cannot be done right now. An excellent strategy to mitigate career obligations is to set scheduled family traditions. Create a Friday night family movie and pizza night. Start a Saturday morning picnic at the park. Treat your kids to breakfast on Sundays. Who doesn't love pancakes? Clearly these and other initiatives are easier to wow a younger child with. Convincing a teenager to attend may take stronger bait, but it can be done. Search for what they like.

My daughter is difficult to please. She isn't afraid to voice her displeasure at a potential family outing. For that reason, I had to search for what she enjoys. I asked questions, paid close attention, and employed the help of my wife and son. I learned that my daughter has two great loves in life: Matcha Latte's and shopping. Although I'm not one for crowds, malls, and shopping, I made it a routine for her and me to grab a drink and hit the shops once per week. Creating this space for your children makes them feel seen and heard. They matter to you. Focus on what they want to do and watch them open up to you. There is nothing like the feeling of your child looking forward to spending time with you. It is a bond that lasts a lifetime.

Remember the minds of children and teens is selfish, so when doing this, always seek to locate the most important priority for them. Doing this will help you identify which of their events are most important and help to prioritize which events are a must to attend. They will be happy when you explain that you are trying to make them a priority and involve them in your decision-making process.

When you attend, you will see them light up in a way you never thought possible. There is no quarterly profit report or increased gains report that can come close to the feeling when you child lights up because you are in the room. Trust me my friend. This is the kind of stuff books are written about!

<u>Superdad Pro-Tips:</u>

1. Set aside time each week to listen to your children.

2. Keep a list of things THEY want to do.

3. Set a schedule to do things THEY want to do each week.

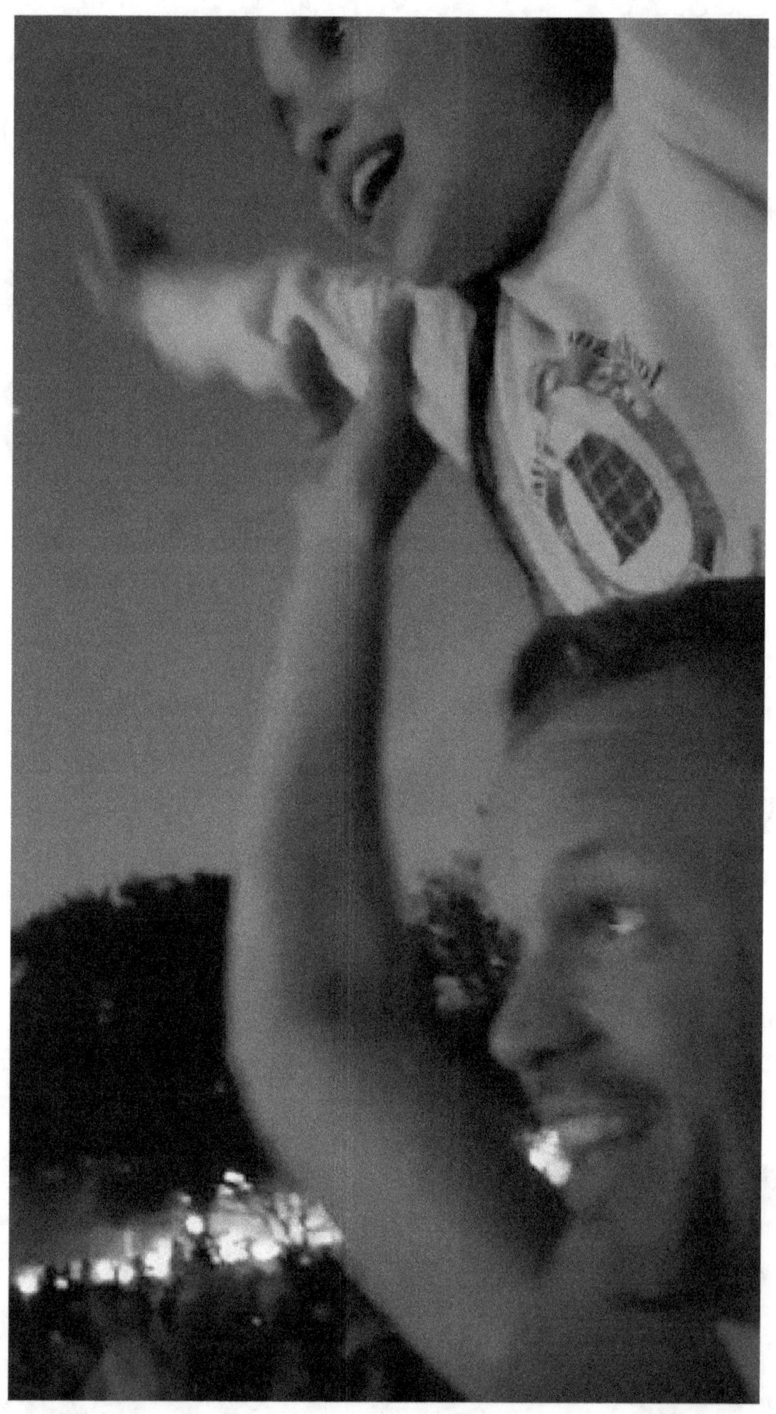

Chapter 2 – Principled

"Important principles may, and must, be inflexible"

-Abraham Lincoln

Ever heard other's opinion of you without their knowledge of your audience? It is quite revealing, isn't it? A confounding thing about relationships is we generally don't say what we really see, think, and feel. We sugar coat the medicine with a softer version of the truth. We do this because we're afraid we might hurt someone else's feelings or worse, they leave the relationship altogether. Fear of loss is a powerful motivation, especially for someone struggling with abandonment issues.

What if we actually told each other the truth? Can you handle your inner circle telling you their honest, unfiltered opinion of your character? What a difference that would be, huh. No more what did he or she mean by that. No more wondering where we stood with individuals. Wouldn't that be refreshing? To say exactly what we think without fear of reaction or rebuttal.

It is so difficult to see your true self the way others see you. It is a tough pill to swallow. When I got sober and quit drinking in 2022 after eleven years of hiding in a bottle, I had to face my feelings for the first time. Nowhere to hide. Nowhere to run. As if that wasn't enough, I also had to face the mess I had made in my relationships, starting at home. Hearing what the people around me saw, heard, felt, and thought almost crushed me. But it was necessary.

You see, many of us, especially addicts, see ourselves through illusory superiority. We think we're doing better than we really are. And it's not just addicts that fall prey to this illusion. Many of the men I speak to don't want to see or hear the truth. They busy themselves, get locked in at work and responsibilities so there is no time for a serious conversation. Avoidance is a powerful weapon.

When the stars align and a conversation is no longer avoidable, they employ gaslighting as a primary defense mechanism. Why are men always on the defensive? We cannot stand quietly and accept another's insights. We are not perfect. We are flawed. No, humility cannot win. We must be tough and fight back. We must ready the cannons. Fire!

My addiction fought hard to stay alive. I'm embarrassed to admit here for all to read that I did everything written in previous paragraphs and more when confronted with truth. My addiction and stubborn pride would not go without a war. But they finally broke because a lie has no endurance. I found my freedom from stubborn pride that kept me sick.

Perhaps you are not dealing with addiction and live a generally blameless life. You're a good man that works hard, raises his children, and never breaks legal or societal norms. You're just looking to improve your parenting skills. You may have a head start in this trait.

This chapter is about locating our principles, or core value system, that will help guide our lives and serve as a lighthouse for our children in a crazy world. We must know and stay glued to these in times of testing and trials. To identify our principles, we must get honest about who we really are.

In my experience, most people (especially men) project a public image that is not close to reality. We puff up our chests, deepen our voices, do a quick set of push-ups backstage, and project the strength we want the world to see. Key and Peele, the acclaimed comedians, illustrate this point in their hilarious short video "Phone Call" where a man ordering ballet tickets changes his tone and demeanor while on the phone because another man next to him. It is an example of how men feel they must posture up and be tough all the time. While it is sarcasm, the skit does point of how insecure we really are.

An authentic, principled man doesn't have to create a false identity or defend himself. His actions speak louder than any appearance or philosophical argument. He doesn't have to fret or feel insecure because he knows exactly who he is and who he isn't. What you do when no one is looking is who you really are. We spend more time trying to create an image when we should focus that energy on being true, authentic, and principled. That is what real men are made of and that is what real women want.

Therefore, honest feedback is so important to principles. We can walk through life lying to ourselves that we are this and that, but not realize we aren't even close in the world's eyes. We must first face what everyone else sees. Only then will we know the truth about ourselves. Only when we take the medicine of honest feedback from trusted loved ones and friends, can we begin to form our core principles.

Here come the defenses. I don't care what anyone else thinks about me. Yes, you do. You own a mirror. You dress yourself. You fix your hair. Oh, you meant you don't care about people's opinions about your character. Then why defend yourself? Why listen to what they said about you? You see, all the bravado and subterfuge are a defense to protect our pride. Along with gaslighting and sarcasm, they serve our purposes to keep every possible threat to our ego at bay.

What a beautiful gift self-honesty is to give your family. No more appearances. No more don't say this or that. Your wife and children will be shocked and probably unsure at first. Don't expect this to work the first time you ask for feedback. But when they realize that you genuinely want to hear what they have to say without defense, your relationship will flourish! It is a gift of freedom for them to speak their truth. It gives your wife and children agency in the family power dynamic. It gives them a voice.

Once we see what everyone else sees, we can take a true inventory of what we are. Only then can we begin to answer the question, what kind of man do I want to be? This is beyond a simple trite definition of a man. What are your qualities? What are the qualities you want to foster in your children? What are the things that matters most to you? Look into the future, twenty years from now, what do you hope your family will say about you? The answer to these questions is probably your principles.

We teach our children two principles in our home: respect and honesty. My stepdad instilled in me and my brother the principle of respecting every adult in every situation. I've expanded that principle to include every person in every situation. We teach our children to be a person that respects the humanity in every person because the Creator made them too, even your enemy.

Respect was defined as fear where I grew up on the westside of Chicago. I can beat you up or worse, so you do what I say. It was such a primitive way of thinking, but it was my reality. And it is for many of the students I work with. Kids need to be taught the definition and value of true respect. Respect for another's rights, property, thoughts, decisions, and speech. This value is not being taught in many homes.

Our children know they have a right to think for themselves. They can formulate their own opinions and others have the same right. No one controls you, nor do you control anyone else. We respect the right of another to disagree with us and are not threatened by it. There is enough room on the planet for conflicting ideas. Sometimes in life it is merely a difference of upbringing or circumstance. Giving someone the freedom to make their own conclusion is empowerment.

Respect means you can disagree with someone and don't have to be enemies. You don't have to resort to ad hominem like a politician in election season. How insecure? When you sink to attacking someone rather than discuss the differing ideas you are revealing how weak your mind is. We generally encourage our children to avoid such people. You don't win an argument by arguing with a fool. You only prove there are two fools in the argument.

True respect is not always easy. People today are angrier and more willing to fight. It seems the entire world has lost impulse control. Teaching your children to respectful in every situation will require much reinforcement, especially when it is adults who do not reciprocate. We encountered such a person during my son's freshmen year in high school.

As long as I can remember Jayden has been in advanced mathematics. He enrolled in one high school where they scheduled him in Honors Algebra 2. He would transfer schools after two weeks and enroll in Honors Geometry at his new school. The geometry teacher decided to give Jayden a test on his first day and count it towards his overall grade. Furthermore, he would have to make up each assignment the class did during the first nine days of class.

No pity parties here. We encouraged Jay to get to work at home, drove him daily at 6:00am to tutoring, and had him re-test. It seemed no matter how hard Jay (and we) worked, Jay's grade only increased incrementally. It appeared there was more than grades and papers going on, but we didn't know what. Then it happened. Jay came home and informed us the teacher got angry with him.

This particular class was second period where the pledge of allegiance and announcements are made. The teacher interrupted the pledge with a directive for the class to be seated and continue working on a bell ringer, but Jay stood and finished reciting the pledge. Jay had directly disobeyed the teacher and felt this meant his grade would suffer. Turns out he wasn't wrong, but we had to make a choice between a number grade and character.

Now we are an extremely unapologetically patriotic family. Countless family members and friends have fought for and died in combat protecting the freedoms that we enjoy. To that end, we honor them by standing, removing our hats, and reciting the pledge of allegiance. This may seem silly or trite to you. Again, we all get to choose our principles in life.

Jayden continued to stand while the pledge continued, much to the displeasure of this teacher. Jay told us he wanted to change teachers because he feels like this teacher has a personal vendetta against him. Fran and I discussed it and concluded that we can't teach Jay to run because he will want to run every time life gets rough. We will continue to do our part with driving him to tutoring, make up appointments, and re-tests. The greater test would be for Jay to show respect in the face of an adult that clearly behaves like a petulant child having their ba-ba taken away.

I'm extremely proud of my son for many things, but this experience is certainly at the top of my list. Jayden continued to walk in the class every other day and greet the teacher with respect despite punishing him via his grade. He never traded barbs or made excuses. Other students in class who rarely turned in homework, skipped class, and never attended tutoring enjoyed higher grades than Jayden. But Jayden remained respectful. You see, hating people is easy to do if you run away. It is hard to grant people their dignity, even when they deprive you of yours. This is a lesson Jayden will never forget. Grades will come and go, but his character is forever.

Fran and I agreed almost two decades ago that honesty is the best foundation of any relationship, especially a marriage and raising children. We started our relationship being honest about our past lives, mistakes, relationships, and shortcomings. It was a painful exercise to go through but seventeen years later I'm so glad we did. Almost all the relationships we've watched over the years that are built on pretentiousness ended badly. It is a fact that we lament. There are very few happily married couples today. For that reason and more, I will begin work on a book that addresses marriage in the coming months when this work is finished. I think I already have a title, "Super" themed.

We decided that if honesty was good for our relationship, then it would be great for our children as well. We have taught our children to tell the truth all the time. Initially children take this point quiet literally and think they must tell you everything that happens. It is so beautiful how innocent the mind of a child is! We must teach our children that we want to know the important facts, the main idea if you will.

As our children have aged, it has become a joy to listen to the important details of their lives. The good and the bad. The greatest challenge in the beginning is to pause your reaction. Listen. Don't react. We dads want to protect our kids. If you grew up in an abusive environment like I did, then this is especially important to you. We can kill our communication by overreacting to what we're hearing. I'm not saying don't do anything about what you're hearing. But not in the moment. Stay still, be present, and just listen. We will address protection in chapter six. As far as you are concerned, just listen for now. Let them develop the trust in you to tell you things that most parents never hear.

This will take time and work. Winning a Superbowl in Chicago seems easier than developing honesty in a teenager. They learn to be deceptive and shifty in elementary school. They hone those skills in middle school. By high school they can graduate to lying to your face without a flinch. The internet has only increased the speed at which these skills are learned. Kids today are facing what we experienced and so much more online.

It may be scary to hear some of the things that happen in schools today, but what is scarier? Hearing the stories or not knowing what your kid is seeing and hearing? I don't know about you, but I'd rather know! Jay and Bella have grown up in a family that doesn't keep secrets. Of course, we celebrated Christmas and told the Santa stories, but no life secrets. They both understand that we are only as sick as our secrets.

This does not mean we deprive our children personal space. In fact, the exact opposite. I do not check my children's phones. I do not listen in on their phone calls. I intentionally give them their space in the same way I value my privacy. I don't have to know everything in my children's lives and probably don't want to. I trust my children to reveal the important details to Fran and me. They know we are the two people on Earth that will not judge them and support them no matter what.

We believe our two principles that we've chosen for our family create strong roots for any relationship. That is what we want to provide our children. Strong roots, healthy roots. I have also created two principles of sobriety for myself: forgive and don't drink. I even got them tattooed on my arms so I will never forget them. I will share more on these in an upcoming book, "My Journey to Sobriety."

Whatever you decide are your principles, be sure of a few things. First, don't have too many. Live Science magazine published an article, "Mind's Limit Found: 4 Things at Once" where the mind appears to have limits on how much it can remember at once. "The Magical Mystery Four: How is Working Memory Capacity Limited, and Why?" published in the National Library of Medicine found those same limits on what our brain can remember.

Remember the goal is to identify the core principles. We can create a list of thousands of valuable lessons for our children, but they won't remember them. We must funnel our core value systems into a few principles that they can assimilate and remember in their adult life. I recommend no more than three.

Second, and most importantly, be sure you live up to the principles you teach. We will talk more about consistency in the next chapter but suffice it to say that nothing will hijack your child's ability to follow your example if you are a hypocrite. Practice what you preach. And when you do fall short, as we all do, own it. Don't run and hide. Be an example for them to follow and watch your child begin to look to you as a leader in their lives. It won't happen overnight, but what great task does? Be patient and stick to your principles. Your child will appreciate the work you've done.

<u>Superdad Pro-Tips:</u>

1. Brainstorm with your spouse about your family principles.

2. Create 2-3 family principles that encompass your values.

3. Share your principles with your children and make them central to decisions.

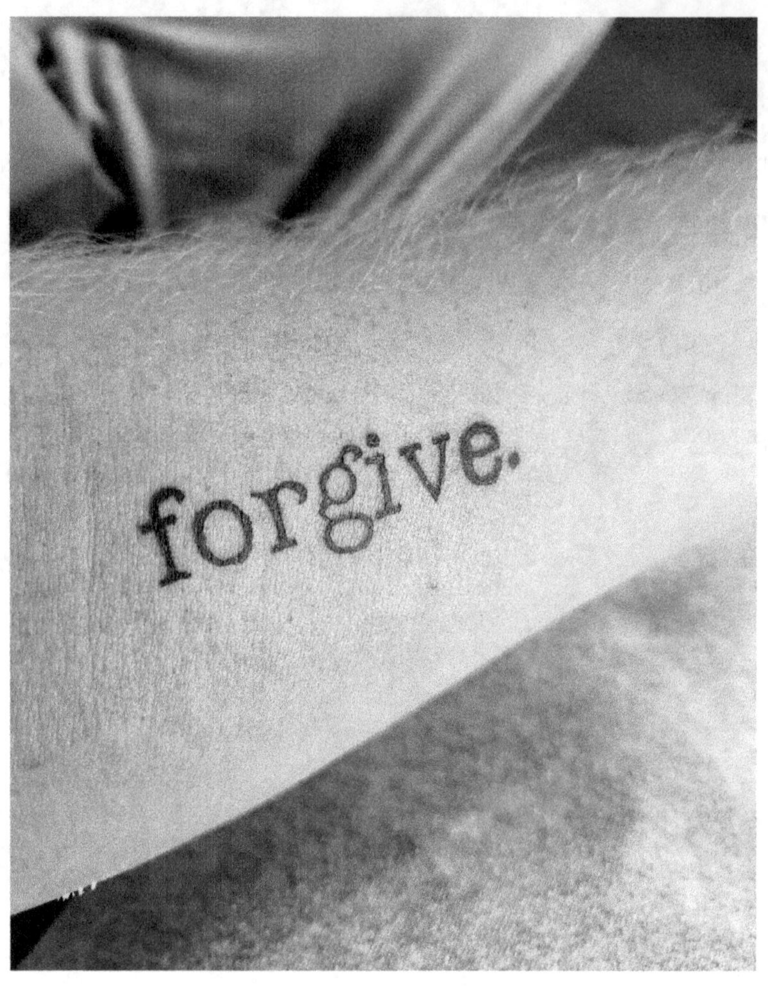
forgive.

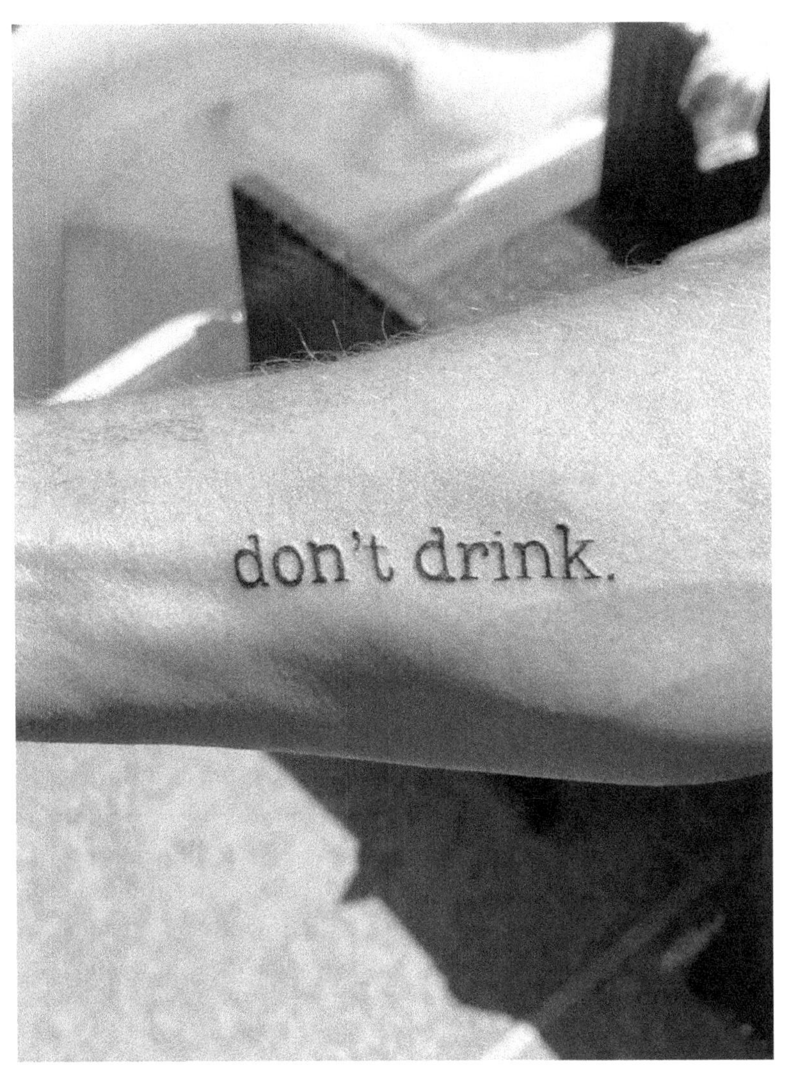
don't drink.

Chapter 3 – Consistent

"Trust is built with consistency"

-Lincoln Chafee

We all want people we can depend on in our lives. You're certain that whether its Monday or Saturday, summer or winter, good times or bad, they're consistent in their character and principles. It is rare these days to find someone who doesn't change according to how things in their day are going. Most American families become mood altering substances for each other. It is dysfunctional co-dependency. If you come home in a bad mood, the entire house must walk on eggshells. Don't upset dad or the rest of the day will be ruined. What a sad existence for a child, or a spouse for that matter.

Children don't get to pick their parents or families. In this sense, they are powerless. They are captive to whatever mood or disposition we are in. Emotional consistency is the glue to your relationship. It is the foundation of trust. How you react should be consistent. We should not be an emotional roller coaster for our children.

In the previous chapter we discussed being a principled man. Hopefully by now you've taken the time to sit, quiet yourself, and listen to the people who know you best on this planet. Identifying and narrowing down your principles means you can begin to teach them to your children. What a beautiful gift, to teach them what we are and what we're not. This gives children an identity in a world gone mad. It is a lighthouse when life gets rough.

Now we must live up to those principles. This is the difficult work. We get to practice what we preach. We must remember that they are watching us. We can discredit our entire message here by living contrary to what we are teaching. Funny thing about teaching principles, it takes a lifetime to teach, but only a moment to tear down.

I'm not suggesting that you must be perfect from now on. Heck no. I mess up more than anyone I can think of. But when I do make mistakes, I own it. I humble myself. No excuse or diatribe. Just genuine remorse and a promise to work harder on it. Remind them you are not perfect. It is this powerful example they will remember. That you too can own you own your mess with explanation or exemption.

Many parents fall into the superiority trap where they believe because they work, pay the bills, and deal with pressures our kids don't even know exist, somehow it gives them permission to ignore this concept of reconciliation. By ignoring this important step, you invite feelings resentment in your children. You create a 'do for thee, not for me' world for them. I don't know about you, but I resent being treated like that. If I ask my wife, children, students, or players to do something then I better be willing to do it equally or harder. But I haven't always been a great example of this concept.

I remember when the children were small, we would take my stepdad out to eat every Tuesday. It is a family tradition, Tuesdays with Carter. The five of us went out to eat at the local Chinese buffet where I would tell the kids to lie about their ages to get a cheaper price. It was only a year I told myself. I remember one such night my daughter spoke up and corrected her age. Bella is just like me, not going to stay quiet.

I'm embarrassed to admit that I got upset. We sat down at the table, and I asked what she thought she was doing? She reminded me of our principles. "We're Schwaegerman's. We don't lie" she said. Wow! She was right! I had to face the truth. I was teaching my kids to lie through my actions while telling them not to. Small or not, it's a lie. If I said here is your favorite meal, but there's one catch. There is a teeny, tiny piece of feces in it. It's just a small piece. You won't even notice it. Microscopic piece. Would you eat it? Of course not! One lie is not acceptable either. We need to remember we are the example. Don't let the poison in.

We went through a very difficult time with my son during his middle school years. That period became known to most as the Covid years, but for us they were the lying years. Jayden kept lying to us. He would lie about superfluous things; he would lie about serious matters. We tried everything. Tough love. Talking. Threats. Nothing seemed to crack him out of this lying phase.

I'll never forget the epiphany I had one morning meditation. While quiet one day it hit me, I was telling kids to be honest while I was lying to myself about my drinking problem. I told myself I had it under control. I'm working full-time, getting paid well, providing. I don't have a problem and even if I do, I'm a functional addict. The only problem with functional addition is your body doesn't know the difference. It still kills you.

I was lying to myself with every bottle of beer right in front of my children but expecting them to tell the truth. I'm dishonest, but they must be honest. What a hypocrite I was! Facing that truth, I immediately called the family together. I looked each one in the eyes and told them of my new realization. It was so painful, yet so freeing. The problem with living a lie is it's exhausting. A lie has no endurance. But the truth will power you through tough times.

Being consistent doesn't mean you will be faultless. It means you will accept truth and humble yourself when you're wrong. So many parents I know worry about image. How will my children look at me if... or what will they think about me? That is no way to live. I'd rather live the rest of my days in an honest relationship that is a rough road than a smooth one paved with lies.

Children are wonderful at forgiveness. Who knows? They may surprise you with their ability to see past your mistakes and may respect you more for the courage it takes to own your stuff. This generation if often criticized for their sense of entitlement and laziness, but no one ever gives them credit for what they're great at, like acceptance and forgiveness. We're the generation that holds grudges and get even.

So, you think you can hide your flaws from your children? News flash! If they are older than elementary school, they already know. We forget how fast kids today are exposed to things. They learn quickly because they're exposed to so much online. You're not hiding anything. You're teaching them to be stubborn and pretentious.

Accept that your perfect image isn't perfect. In fact, owning your mess will probably improve the way they see you in the long run. Children are just like us, they want authentic, real relationships. How can we expect them to have honest relationships in their adult lives if we can't have honest conversations with them as children?

Consistency doesn't just extend to our principles and reconciliation. As fathers, we should be consistent in our application of rules and punishment too. This is particularly important when your children are young. Creating a home where children know what the expectations are and what happens when they are broken. We cannot overreact one day and then overlook the next. This is worse than having any rules at all.

This sort of inconsistency encourages a tone-deaf child who will not respect authority or boundaries. It is counterproductive. Now not every infraction requires a nuclear response. But a response, an acknowledgement is necessary here. A rule was broken and is duly noted by your wife and self.

Manipulative kids will try their best to wear you down. They keep at it, looking for a break in your defenses. It is important to be consistent, but also to prioritize. Therefore, identify and keeping principles is so important. You cannot possibly try to enforce every single offense, like some sort of prison warden. Besides, who wants to do that? No parent wants to run around enforcing rules all day, every day.

Your spouse and you should create two levels of offences. A tiered system if you will. Major and minor. What is absolutely not acceptable versus what are just behaviors that kids do. This will help you to major on the majors and minor on the minors. It ensures the punishment fits the crime. That is one of our Constitutional guarantees under the 8th amendment. How much more then should it be afforded to our most precious commodity, our children?

Think about it. How much of our energy is gobbled up by petty, minor offenses? We spend so much time as parents chasing our tails. We neglect the serious matters because by the time we get to them, we're exhausted. Perhaps that's the plan. We must employ an intelligent strategy to be consistent in all areas of raising our children, especially our non-negotiables.

Nothing will discredit your children's trust in you than inconsistency. It's poison to relationships. Many times, we're inconsistent because of convenience. We're too tired, have too much going on at work, or just are worn down by the issue at hand. We must remind ourselves that by giving in now we will pay later. We will be encouraging the behavior to persist, making our future days more stressful.

Why kick the can down the road? Make up your mind that you are going to be consistent. Next time one of your major rules are broken, address it. Next time one of your children points out your mistake, own it. Be consistent in your distribution of punishment and follow through with it. Lying should be met with the same punishment each month. It shouldn't receive a one month ban from Xbox in August but get one day in October.

Let's be consistent in our rewards as well. I mention in chapter 8 that we pay our children for daily and weekly chores. We also pay for grades. We believe in rewards as many to a desired result of behavior. We should be consistent there too. Consistency quiets all the voices of doubt and cynicism that seek to discredit your parenting. By creating paydays, we celebrate the kid's hard work. They get to reap the rewards of their consistent efforts. It is a symbiotic relationship.

Consistency is a must in you are going to teach your children anything. Robert Marzano, a leading educational researcher opined that it takes seven encounters with new information for that concept to become long-term memory. Most rehabilitation clinics understand and operate on the twenty-eight-day rule, where it takes as long to break old habits and create new ones in their place.

These realities prove the need for consistency in parenting. We are teachers. We teach breaking bad habits and creating new ones. No faking here. How can we create consistent habits in our children if we are engaged in bad habits? I've met parents that attempt this. Heck, I was one! The result is generally worse than if any leadership was asserted at all. Children spot fake immediately. They are allergic to it.

Please hear me Superdads...before you jump into some of these techniques, take the time to get quiet and listen. Be sure you aren't creating a hinderance by ignoring your own stuff while expecting your children to own theirs. Nothing could be more self-sabotaging. I like to start every new conversation about my children by opening and humbling myself. Talking about times I screwed up or blew it. This sort of self-deprecation can serve your purposes of parenting well.

You see, our children hold us in high regard, whether they admit it or not. They look up to us. We fed and cleaned them when they couldn't do it for themselves. No matter how many mistakes you've made in your child's life, they still want to hear your humility. It is so refreshing to them. It takes you off the pedestal and humanizes you to them. What a gift! Humility!

And why is that so hard for us men? We're taught from an early age…don't cry. Don't show emotion. Always project strength. Problem with that approach is it's hard to get close to someone that always has defenses up and on high alert. There is a better way. Instead of chasing perfection, we should aim to foster the desire to stick to it. Explain how you've blown it. Make that less scary. Getting rid of the fear of failure removes the stigma from trying.

If you've ever dealt with performance anxiety, then you know how crippling it can be. Our children don't want to let us down. But they're going to do just that. They will fail, fall short, and blow it too. We must remove the stinger of falling short. Negative consequences never made anyone a better person, just compliant. We should provide positive rewards and support when our child does mess up. It isn't the end of the world. It's just a mistake. Start being consistent again today.

This freedom and acceptance creates a world for them that isn't so scary to try and accept their own humanity because you did. When you humble yourself in your child's eyes, you give them permission to try and fail and try again. And that is consistency. Is it not? Refusing to quit trying. I refuse to quit trying to be a Superdad for my children. They deserve my attempt today.

Superdad Pro-Tips:

1. Seek constructive criticism without defending yourself.

2. Journal your emotional reactions and punishments.

3. Remember to major on the majors, minor on the minors.

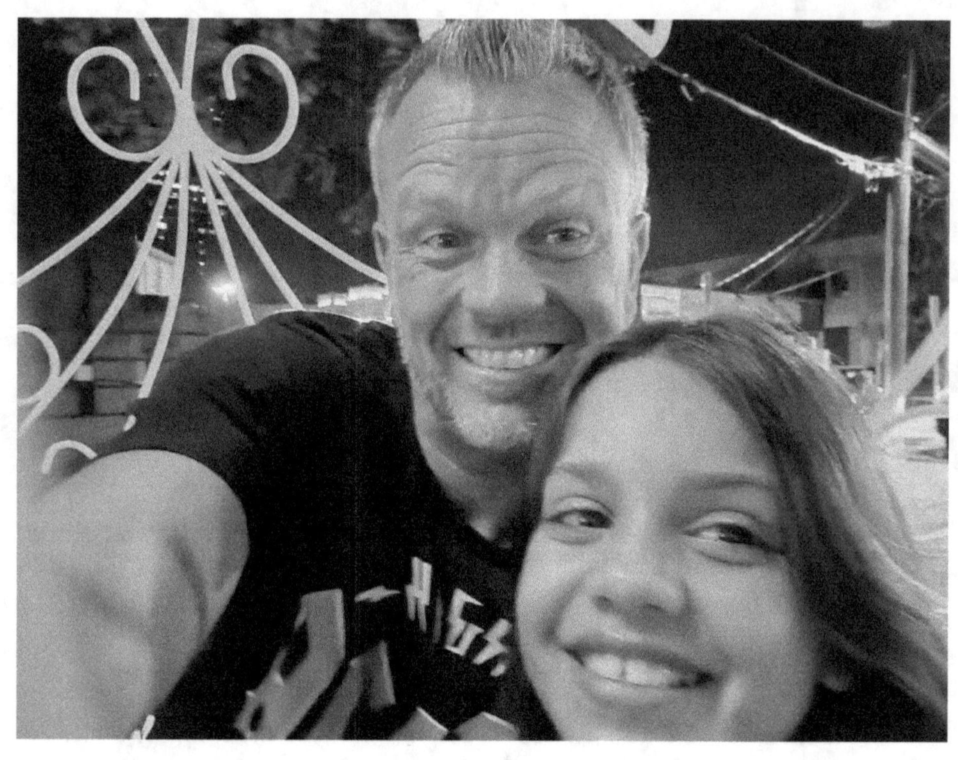

Chapter 4 – Empathic

"Remember what it is like to be a teenager"

-Sadir Karandikar

We are not perfect parents, and we were not parented perfectly. We now understand and empathize with our parents now that we ourselves are in that role. Each generation has difficulty relating to the next, but this generation has significant differences that make it a unique challenge for us parents today.

For starters, the internet has transformed the world as we know it. If you were born before 1980, you remember a life before cell phones, social media, and the invasiveness of the internet. Today's child doesn't know a world without cell phones and internet. They are digital natives, meaning they never knew a paper-based world that we grew up in.

As a teacher, I hear parents mention this all time at parent-teacher conferences. Mostly complaints that their child doesn't care about anything but their phones and being on them. Now I don't pretend to have a magic wand that will poof away a teenage desire to stare mindlessly for hours and days into a 5-inch device without any cares at all. Again, this illustrates my point. This wasn't even a concern for our parents. In this sense, they had it easy compared to us. The world they lived in and raised us in was a much simpler one.

While the world we were raised in might have been a simpler one, it wasn't perfect either. Our parents weren't perfect. Instead of whining about how bad this generation is, perhaps we would be better served to look at some strategies to reach them. With each criticism and each comparison, all we do is drive a wedge of separation between us.

Isn't the goal to form a bond of closeness with our children, not alienate them? Well, let me ask you, do you like being compared to others and criticized? Doesn't feel good, does it? Whether in relationships, career, or our day to day lives, we generally avoid people and situations like this. How would we feel if the next date night our spouse began comparing us to previous relationships? We'd be out of there quick. Why would we think our children would be any different?

Maybe the answer isn't turning back the clocks to the good old days where everything looked and sounded familiar. Perhaps we need to put putting aside our judgements and accept our children are different. They are different because they are growing up in unique times. There are problems kids deal with today we never imagined while playing hide and seek outside. Now kids are being taught to hide from an active shooter.

And different doesn't automatically equal bad or inferior. After all, you may be different too if you were brought up in this generation with technology. We won't ever know what it is like to grow up with the temptations they do because we relied on landlines and prayed parents didn't pick up when we called.

Kids today are faced with so much more at such an earlier age than we ever imagined. Consider a student being bullied or peep pressured at school. Forty years ago, that student came home to a reprieve. They got a break from the bully. Today's students get home, opens their phone, and has messages, alerts, notifications all reminding them how uncool they are. Their bullying doesn't end when the key hits the door lock.

Before I start to sound like an apologist for gen z, please understand my goal here. If we are the adults, shouldn't we set aside our judgements so we can reach our children? Isn't that our goal? We cannot be so stubborn to expect everything to look our way. They are not us. They didn't grow up like us. Giving them this gift of understanding will free them to be the person they can be. How can I be so sure? Because I was the worst example of tearing down this generation and I changed my behavior too. I had to change my behavior habits before my children would ever open up and communicate.

You see, I have been a public high school educator for twenty-one years. I've seen students, hairstyles, fashions, lingo, and fads come and go. I've seen words change meanings. A cap used to be something you put on your head, now it's a lie. No cap. One thing has never changed over these years, and that is a teenagers need to feel heard.

What a powerful thing, to be heard? How many of us visit therapist's and counselor's offices each week to fill this need? I have a friend who is a licensed therapist. We talk about everything under the sun, from politics to sports. He would always say to me, "my profession wouldn't be necessary if people actually listened, heard, and validated each other."

And it is a need. Now you may have been raised like I was, old school. Crying is for the week. Feelings are to be ignored. Never show them where to stick the knife. Yeah, yeah, yeah, tough guy stuff. But we're talking about OUR children here! They didn't get to pick who their parents are. They have no power in that sense. They are stuck. Shouldn't we want more for our kids?

Empathy is the key to unlock conversation with your child. Without conversation, you do not have a relationship. You merely bark commands, to which they comply for monetary provisions or simply to avoid World War 3. Do this and that and I'll give you some money at the end of the week. That is no relationship. That's employment. They are your employee. There is so much more than having a transactional, employee relationship with your kid.

I remember when my son was in middle school and played for the basketball team. He was skilled, but not the most athletic player on the team. As a former player and coach, I felt some obligation to help him improve. You know us dad's love to live vicariously through our children. I'm embarrassed to look back at how immature I was as a competitive parent.

I would show him workouts, exercises, and drills to help him improve. And then we would go to his games and not see much if any improvement. I became frustrated. I took it personally. He doesn't realize how much knowledge I have and how many players I've made better. It was a blow to my ego. How could I go from coaching high school teams to success but not make my son better?

Middle school ended and he got accepted into a wonderful collegiate program where he would earn an associate degree while attending high school. This meant he was leaving all his friends who attended the magnet program pathway and starting new. Fran and I both thought this was his opportunity to really grow. At that age, sometimes friends and peers can keep you stuck. We both agreed we wanted him to go to this new school and start new.

The new school had a summer basketball camp. We didn't miss a day. Each day, I would ask how he felt about the camp and got less than excited, short, one-word answers. How did practice go? Fine. What did you guys work on? Hoop. My assumption was that he was still pouting about missing his friends. I had no idea what was coming next.

School started and Jayden seemed to be adjusting to the classes well. He liked most of his teachers, but when I asked about basketball, he would get quiet and withdrawal. Again, red flag that mom and I chalked up to missing his friends. We learned on the second day of school that the coach was going to hold tryouts. This meant coach was only keeping ten freshmen, so thirty of the forty students in basketball were going to be cut. 25% acceptance rate. Geez, even UT Law has higher acceptance rate than that!

The second week of school came, and our anxieties rose. We knew how much this meant to our son. Then it happened. On the ninth day of school, we learned that Jayden had been cut. To say he was devastated would be an understatement. It was the first time as a father that I was truly worried about the mental health of my kid. He didn't want to talk. He didn't really come out of his room. I felt so powerless to help my son. If there was ever a time in my life that I wanted a magic wand, it was then.

I decided to email the coach and inquire about why Jay was cut. As a former coach, I understand every parent wants to see their child succeed. I was not in any way challenging. I merely asked what he felt are the things Jay can do to improve. What I got back later that day was a blistering three-page, multi-bulleted rebuke highlighting all Jay's deficiencies. I was so angry! Who does this guy think he is? Why would a coach try to crush a kid's spirit like that? Not realizing at the time, that I had also been part of the problem.

Later that night, after debating in my head, I decided to show Jay the email. We don't keep secrets in our family. He sat quietly as we went over the bullets. I asked him what he thought, and his reply shook me to my core. You see, I routinely reminded Jay of the same deficiencies as a motivation to work on them. I pointed out everything he wasn't good at, where he could improve, thinking I was helping. Jay looked up at me and said, "well, I've been told by everyone I'm the slow kid on every team I've played for."

Watching my son begin to cry, I fought back my tears. He went on to describe coaches, teammates, and students who would tease him, call him fat, tell him he is the most "unathletic player" on the team. I hugged him tight and apologized for hurting him and being part of the problem. We cried while my mind spiraled! I had no idea he was taking a beating all day, only to come home to Mr. Coach who kept the put downs coming. How could I be so blind?

You see, if we don't humble ourselves and empathize with our children, they will never trust us with the deep stuff. Do you open up to people without trust? It is the foundation of communication. If you're doing all the talking that isn't communication. I did a terrible job of creating an environment where my children felt that no matter what they told me, I would understand, or seek to understand. No judgement. No "I told you so's" but real empathy that validates their feelings and existence.

I'm so happy to say that a year later my son and I are in a much better place because of this. We talk everyday about our feelings, challenges, hopes, and dreams. We both became vegetarians for different reasons. He asked me to train him daily. He even joined a select traveling team through the urging of a friend that has taught him so much and brought us to different cities across America. He is now entering his sophomore year as a varsity basketball player at another high school. I couldn't be prouder of the growth of our relationship and his mindset.

We dad's need to remember that we are the leader. That does not mean barking orders. It means we should be leading by example. Next time we get a case of the "I told you so's" we should be reminded that it only separates us from our goal of connectivity with our children. Put yourself in their shoes before you charge in. Take a moment to remember how you wanted to be treated and remember it's alright to just listen. You don't have to always answer. Remember, if you're the only one talking, that isn't communication. And always keep at the center what is truly important: your relationship with your child.

Let's prioritize making our children feeling heard and validated. Start by simply asking them open-ended questions and let them take it from there. Your job is to be present. As a starter, try rephrasing what you hear them say. Oh man, that must have hurt. Oh wow, that must have made you feel amazing. Or how did that make you feel? Don't jump in. Don't take over. Just listen and watch the magic happen.

Do not be surprised if it takes some time. This will require you to employ trait #3 by being consistent. When the conversation begins to flow, acknowledge their feelings about whatever it is they're describing. Young people feel so ignored. They do not feel heard. Do not take what is said as a problem to solve. It is a gift to you. Just acknowledge what they are saying and feeling.

As your child begins to grow in trust and begins to feel validated you may be surprised what they are willing to share. Kids today are extremely lonely. Most adults are too, for that matter. Yes, I know your child may many friends, have a seemingly large online presence, and be on a team, but how many of those people does your child trust and moreover, how many listen?

Most kids perform for each other. Most adults do too, for that matter. We all wear a public mask. We project how we want to be seen, never really facing how we feel, think, experience. This performance trap is such a heavy burden. This too can rob you and your children of a genuine relationship. Forget appearances. People are so fickle anyway. Love you one moment, turn on you the next. Try to make you child feel as though they can say anything, and it stays there with no judgement. By creating this space for you and your child to just be, you are paving a road to be a part of the good stuff in their lives.

Try and remember how much road is ahead in your kid's life. It isn't always about what is going on right here and now. Keep the end game in mind. Whatever stage your kid is at, there is more to come. Much more. Games, practices, dates, break-ups, proms, graduation, moving, college, jobs, marriage, kids of their own. We want to be a part of these events and benchmarks, not just an afterthought.

Our children will want to talk to us before making decisions because of the trust we formed through empathy. Why? Because we took the time to patiently, consistently prove that they are safe, telling us about their life is safe. It still shocks me to this day when my son asks my opinion. I spent so many years trying to cram mine down his throat and now he comes to me. It is astonishing how well this works if you make understanding them and leaving your judgment at the door.

Now this is not a microwave solution. You cannot expect to be Mr. Cram down your throat for 13 years and just because you listened once that all is well. That's a bit naïve. To put it in coaching terms, you must establish good habits for the bad ones to dissipate and eventually disappear. We can't allow ourselves to be focused on getting a result in the beginning. It will come. Be patient. Just listen. What do you lose by listening and validating you child?

<u>Superdad Pro-Tips:</u>

1. Create a list of questions to get your kids talking about their school, day, friends, interests, etc.

2. Set a scheduled "teach dad" time where they can inform you.

3. Remember, don't interrupt, or interject, just ask questions, and let them talk.

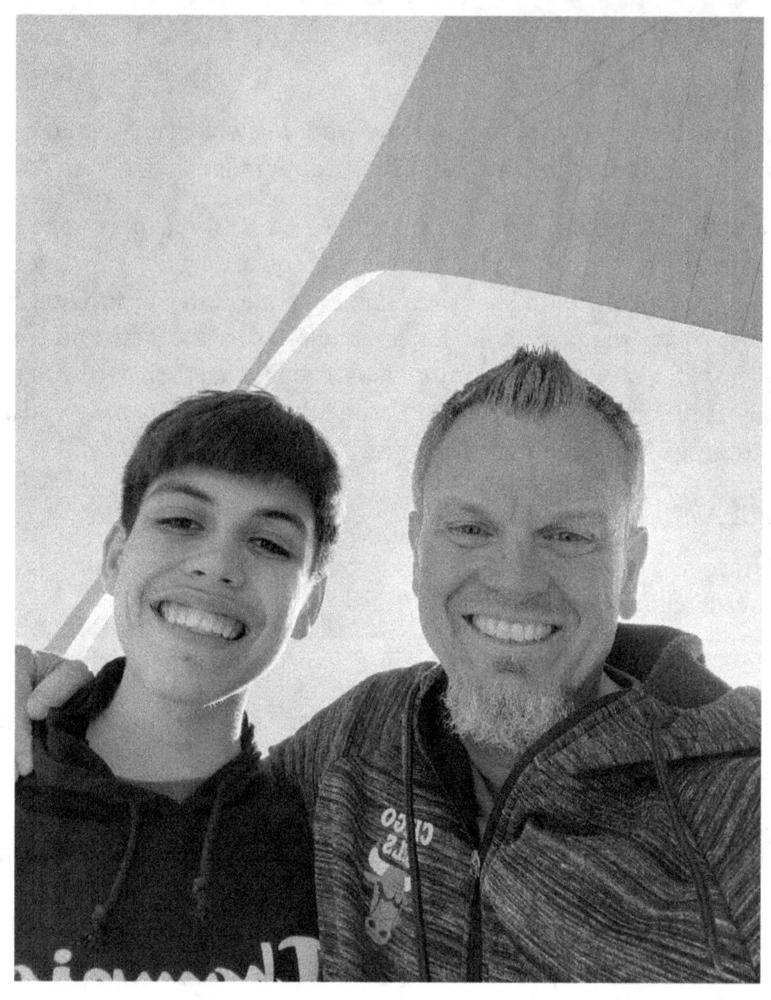

Chapter 5 – Encouraging

"True teachers use themselves as bridges over which they invite their students to cross; then, having facilitated their crossing, joyfully collapse, encouraging them to create bridges of their own"

-Nikos Kazantzakis

Don't we all love people that make us feel as if we can do anything? We will take direction from them. We will run through a brick wall for them, or at least get a headache trying. Why? Because they prove they believe in us by giving us the power to do something and the freedom to mess up. Encouraging Superdads go beyond saying I believe in you. They show it. Allowing children to make decisions and take risks is what being an encouraging Superdad is all about.

Empowerment for children is so important. Never do anything for them that they can do for themselves, an old friend of mine used to say. Many controlling parents feel a need to have everything perfect, or at least what they perceive as perfect. Fran and I both are perfectionists. I can relate to the words of late US Senator John McCain's daughter said of him at his funeral, "he was a perfectionist and couldn't understand why everyone else wasn't."

We both grew up in homes that had high expectations for tasks and were expected to measure up. When things weren't done correctly, there was hell to pay. We learned it was easier to it right the first time, than to give half effort and must do it over again...not to mention what emotions might come with that displeasure. We assimilated this perfect complex and started raising our children under the same. We both continued the pattern of micro-management, almost looking for the wrong so we can swoop in and do it for them.

How many parents do this? We get frustrated because they don't care about cleaning, or some random tasks. Well, of course they don't care about cleaning a house they didn't have to work and pay for. The key here is to empower by giving the task and allowing them to do it. Not done correctly? They do it again, not you. There is nothing wrong with a little quality control. But there is a bigger issue at hand. We must learn to let go.

We must begin preparing, truly preparing, our kids for independent adult life. Sometimes we parents want to do too much for our kids that they can do. We are enabling adult children by helicoptering our kids. And they learn to take advantage fast. Our kids aren't stupid. They see that if they just don't do something to our liking, we will swoop in and do it for them.

To put things in a larger context, what about choices in your teen's life? What school they attend, what team they play on, who their friends are, who they date, their curfew, and on. You see, many of these choices you will little to no power to control. You may think you have power, but when kids get on a bus or step out of the car at drop-off, they are in control. And what happens in school may surprise and shock you.

Let's take the rosy colored glasses off and accept that we aren't perfect parents, therefore, our kids aren't perfect either. We need to prioritize our focus and efforts on what we really believe is critical. For Fran and I that is education. We believe that if there is one area that we cannot allow our children to fail, it is learning. After all, we believe that is the key to a successful life in an ever-changing world and economy.

That is not to say that we completely neglect the other areas of our children's lives, but we give them space and freedom. We focus our parental energy on education. We check grades. We email teachers. We have a 'homework first' policy. We reward success. We punish failure. One could say when it comes to education, we are all up their business. We decided that if there is one area we will not fail, it is education.

Perhaps it's because I've worked in education for over two decades. Perhaps it's because Fran and I both grew up in urban, public schools and know what is out there. Whatever the motivation, failure is not an option for our children. We understand that our children need room to make choices, but some things are not important to the mind of a child until it is too late, like education.

Kids today are conditioned to immediate gratification. Post the right video, get clicks, likes, loves, comments and your need to feel important, significant are met almost immediately. You can become almost instantly viral. That seems to be all kids dream today, to make the video that gets them famous. They fantasize about being famous, as if that will fix all their problems at once. What they don't realize is how many new problems show up with fame and fortune.

They are not familiar with delayed gratification. Working hard at something for years. Being patient for your opportunity. We needed to make education a priority because society doesn't place much importance on it anymore. Being an educated person will always help you. Whether you become a famous Youtuber or just work in a skilled job, education will keep you grounded. You will never reach a point in your life when you regret being an educated person. You will probably have regrets in your life, but that will not be one of them.

How does all this tie together? We need to communicate to our children what our focus is for them and that we will 'back off' other areas. We will give them some of the power they crave in social areas of their lives. We will trust them. All we ask in return is to take on the area of focus and communicate. This is really a strategic move on our part. You see, we don't *really* have any power to give, but they don't know that. This is about fostering a trust relationship with your child. We're giving them choice.

I remember when Jayden was cut from his basketball team in the second week of his freshmen year. As we discussed in chapter 4, Jayden was in a remarkable Early College program that Fran and I genuinely loved. However, we listened to Jayden's request to transfer to a Magnet school where his middle school friends attended, and he would be given a try-out for the basketball team. This was a huge ask, since this is the same friend group from middle school when we went through the lying phase.

Fran and I talked it over and after a sleepless night, we decided to trust Jayden. We would grant his request and change schools. He was so happy. We both explained to him in our own way that this is HIS decision. We were empowering him to make a choice about his life. What happens next is a direct reflection on him and his decisions. We had no guarantee this would work out. Friends tried to ensure us that we were doing what is best, but as a parent you always question yourself.

It is a remarkable thing to watch your child succeed on their own. Jayden did just that. He earned honor roll all four report cards and was even inducted into the National Honor Society after his Freshmen year. We never know what our kids can do if we always do it for them. It is scary. Letting go of power is hard. Even if that power is fiat. It is our minds that want to control all the variables in our children's life as if we can manipulate the universe to be kind to them.

Absolutely not. Truth is we have no power. Helicopter parents only create adult children. Kids grow into bigger kids. They cannot make decisions for themselves. They cannot deal with failure. I've always told Jayden and Bella to try new moves in practice. Living at home is practice for real life. Make your mistakes in practice. There you have support. You can work to improve before the lights are on. Whether it's basketball or dance or drama, try new moves in practice. We must allow our kids to try new moves at practice.

We went through something similar with Bella and her schooling at an early age. Our local elementary school converted into a Montessori school after Bella's Kinder year. Bella would have to test high enough to get admitted into the program. She scored high enough to be admitted and attended for one year. She did not like the program. She felt like she was being used as a tutor, or sorts, for other students in lower grade levels.

We discussed other options for her schooling, and she chose a performing arts school in a rougher part of the district. At first, Fran and I didn't like the idea since the school was roughly ten miles from our home and that meant Bella would have to ride the bus. We also weren't thrilled with the neighborhood the school was located. But Bella insisted this was where she wanted to be, so we made it happen.

Again, we empowered our children to communicate what they wanted for their education. We listened, considered, weighed the pros and cons, and ultimately decided to trust our Bella's instincts. We explained to her that this would be her decision and a reflection on her character. I'm so proud to say that she flourished in that school, learning to act, play piano, and speak Spanish in addition to mastering the basic four core areas of learning. She loved her time there. But it wouldn't have happened without trusting our kids.

How do I start, you ask? I recommend starting with a conversation with your spouse. Make sure you are both on the same page about what is a priority in your kids' lives. This way you aren't stepping on each other in the process. Decide what areas you will be tight and loose on. This may take some time as you may have grown up differently, with different parenting styles. Fran and I grew up with an emphasis on family responsibilities like cleaning, looking after younger siblings, babysitting, etc. Grades and school were a distant second, at best. That is something we both agreed would be a priority for our children.

Next step is to communicate with your children exactly how you will empower them. Explain when you will check their progress and what metrics you will us to judge. This all needs to be pre-established between parents. Communication is key. It doesn't matter what it is, communication will be the major factor in how well it works out. We're not simply talking about communicating once. Empowerment means we trust you and in return you trust us. You take the controlling hands off and your kids tell you what is really going on. It is a symbiotic relationship. The more you do your part, the more they feel confident to do theirs. Others might call it a win-win relationship.

Lastly, and most importantly, when they do mess up don't freak out. It will happen. It is how they learn. Some parents try to steer their children away from experiencing any failure. It must be exhausting. And what does it teach the kid? That they will never fail in life? Oh please. Life is full of failure. It's what you do afterwards that makes a winner. John Maxwell in his book *Failing Forward* said, "It's not what happens to me; it's what happens in me. It's not the size of the problem, but how I handle the problem. When I fall, keep getting up."

President Theodore Roosevelt said, "He who makes no mistakes makes no progress." Why do we work so hard to keep our kids from falling and skinning their knee? Failure is inevitable. Success and failure are not a percentage, test, or event. They are a process. Because in life the question isn't if you will have problems and fail. The question is how you will react. Encouraging Superdads know this and support their children to foster a positive attitude towards success *and* failure. It's not about a score. It is about developing the right attitude. Success will chase down people who have the right attitude and we must encourage that in our children for them to achieve more than we ever dreamed.

<u>**Superdad Pro-Tips:**</u>

1. Choose one idea your child has wanted and completely support it without judgement.

2. Do not offer advice. Wait for them to ask for your input.

3. When the ask for input, support their effort, not the result.

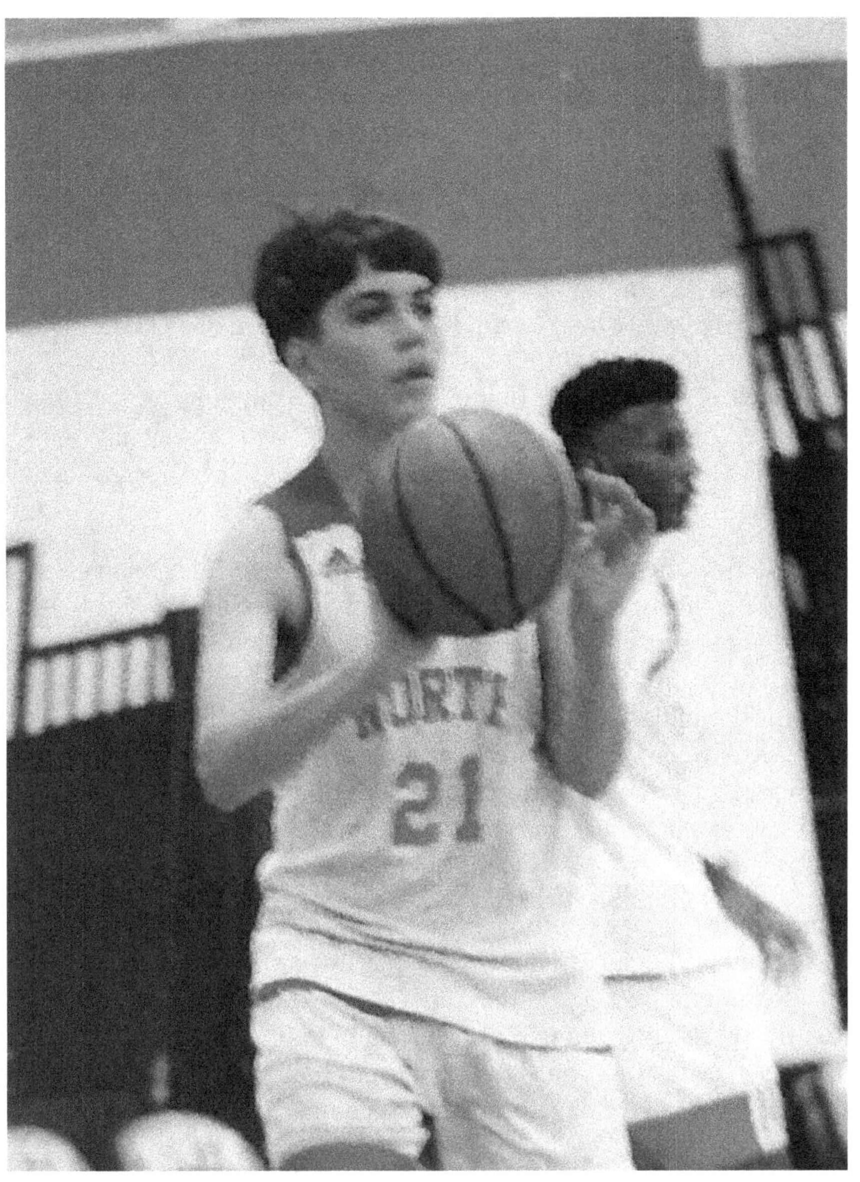
NORTH
21

Chapter 6 – Protective

"I cannot think of any need in childhood as strong as the need for a father's protection"

-Sigmund Freud

What is protection? To the mind of a small child protection is such a simple thing. Pick me up when I fall and scrape my knee. Hold me when I get stung by a bee. As children grow up, protection takes on a new curve for parents. At first, we do everything. We feed, bath, and even wipe their behinds for them. They can't do anything for themselves. As they age, we let go a little more each passing day. Technology has changed the timeline of innocence, but we have always strived to let our kids be kids if possible.

There is a fine line for parents of teenagers between being an over-protective, helicopter parent and a protective Superdad. Over-protective parents want to do everything, manipulate every variable, and in doing so cripple their children from learning problem solving and critical thinking skills on their own. This sort of relationship fosters resentment in the teen because they're constantly infantized and treated as if they're incompetent. I can think of nothing more destructive to the confidence of a developing young adult.

I have worked in a high school for over two decades and taught seniors for most of my career. Senior year is a stressful transition year for student and parent alike. Many of the parents I talk to describe having difficulty in letting go, and this is especially true of firstborn children. Years fly bye! To go from wiping a behind to letting a child drive themselves to college is hard for any parent to deal with. But it is in that letting go that we develop a stronger bond than ever.

Early years are easy to be a protective Superdad. Just be there. You don't even have to have all the answers. Just be there. Your presence alone can fix most of what ails a small child. But a teenager to young adult seek to become independent. They don't need you as much, or at least they don't want to admit it. Letting go means we are 1) empowering them to make decisions (chapter 5) and 2) being there when it doesn't go as planned, without judgment. Chapters five and six are inseparable in that sense. We must let go for them to seek our advice and protection.

It is this test of the closeness of our relationship that scares parents. What if they don't call or tell me what's going on? What if they cut me off? It is frightening to let go! There are no guarantees in life, but we do know one day we will leave this Earth. We all hope to live a long, healthy life and be with our families for decades. I dream of being a grandparent, spoiler in chief, and grey-haired advisor.

We must prepare of young adults for adult life by letting them make decisions for themselves. When they fail, we must reserve our judgements and quit our "I told ya so's" so they can feel comfortable failing and coming to us. Otherwise, why would they want to? If every half-bad decision is met with an "I told ya so" lecture and scolding, why would they want to tell you? They'll avoid the condemnation and keep it to themselves. Wouldn't you?

Creating this environment doesn't encourage failure, it makes failure less scary and allows them to grow from it. We discuss our failures in our home. Some are more willing participants than others, but we are all a work in progress. We eliminate the fear or shame by discussing what we were thinking and how we can do better next time. We teach that failing doesn't make you a failure. It is a process, not an event. Approaching failure this way means everyone learns the lesson from one failure, rather than all four family members repeating the same.

Our responsibility is to prepare our children for failure and success. Both are a necessary course to graduate the school of adolescence. Helicopter parents only prepare their children for success. This way, the young adult is totally unprepared for the challenges that lie ahead. What will they do when their marriage faces trouble? Turn to helicopter. What will happen when they have troubles at work? Turn to helicopter. They will have no compass from which to navigate the challenges of life on their own. They will always think they need a helicopter.

It is impossible to ask a teenager to share their worst decisions in front of the entire family at the beginning of trying this approach. Nothing is more important to them than their image and they will protect it at all costs. They will spend 12 hours per day promoting their image online.

Rather, start one-on-one. Let them talk. When they begin telling you about failure, don't interrupt, interject, be a dad, or have the answer. Just listen. If you're not sure what to say at any moment, simply ask the question, "how did that make you feel?" That is my go-to when I'm stuck.

You see, we're creating an environment for our kids to tell us about nearly anything. We want to be protective Superdads, but they want to be independent. Secretly they want our advice and support, but we must swallow our pride first. We must stop rushing in and trying to fix them. Just create the safe environment for them to share their failure. This opens the door for so much more than you thought possible.

We cannot and will not be able to stop every bad thing in their lives, but we help them grow from mistakes, so they don't repeat them. We must get out of the mindset that we can superman every harmful thing away from our children. Especially if you come an abusive background as I do, we are prone to over-protection. We know the pain that is out there, and don't want our kids to feel one bit of it.

My perspective of protection was so skewed from early childhood. My biological father emotionally, physically, and sexually abused me. My stepfather was a drill sergeant who sent the message, 'don't bother me'. My mother worked 12-hour night shifts, 6 days per week as a trauma nurse. I was essentially left alone to navigate adolescence and teenage years. What did I do? Fight my own battles. I kept everything to myself. It wasn't until I woke up in a hospital with amnesia that my parents found out I had joined a gang.

My violent and abusive background hurt my ability to shut off the over-protective parent complex because I had a savior complex. I would rush in and try to fix everything. I didn't want my children to experience one ounce of pain. I now know cognitively that this is totally unavoidable as life would have it. At the time, it was a driving emotional force in my life. I remember dropping my kids off at school for the first days and feeling so helpless. I almost couldn't function at work as my every thought shifted back to their well-being.

I remember a phone conversation with Fran while leaving work one day. My son was in elementary school at the time and was jumped on the way to school. Three boys decided to make my son a target and beat him up. Fran knew me well enough to wait until the day was finished to make me aware. At the time, I was most assuredly not mature enough to handle that sort of violent act towards my son.

She had already gone up to the school, talked with the principal, and taken Jay home for the rest of the day. I was blithely unaware, teaching in my high school. My school day ends roughly two hours after my son's elementary school does, but that didn't stop me from driving straight to his school. Only a janitor was on campus as it was late in the evening. I called and left voicemails. I emailed. I wanted vengeance. I grew up with violence. That is why we purchased a home in a suburb twenty outside the city limits. I didn't want my children to go through what I had to.

Once I got home, I asked for the entire story. Turns out Jay had a disagreement at recess the day prior with one of the three boys. That boy went to get two of his older cousins to beat Jay up. Can you hear the helicopter coming? I had failed to protect my son. He suffered and I wasn't there. I failed. I spent the rest of the evening teaching my son wrestling and jiu-jitsu moves so he can defend himself. It was something he clearly didn't want to do. Jay is not a fighter. He is a great kid. He has been taught to fight with his intelligence and wit, not fists.

Looking back at that decision, I wish I made more maturity. I wish I saw the bigger picture of protection. All I communicated to my son is that he is never going to share anything that happens at school again. He would rather avoid the mess at home. My immaturity caused him even more pain later that evening. How could I be so foolish? The most important thing is to keep open lines of communication. Will he come to me next time? No way. I taught Jayden to stuff down any future events at school or in his personal life.

Can you see how dangerous that is? We must get out of our heads that being a Superdad means we protect our children from all pain. That isn't realistic and doesn't help them mature. It is so important to start now. Start small. Try to create an environment of openness in communication with your children. The earlier you start to create this environment, the easier this will be down the road. We need the practice too. They are sharing the worst of their secret failures and we are practicing accepting that our children will fail.

It is precisely that fear that holds us in captive to the controlling parent role. Break that fear. Walk in the light that the most important thing for your child is to trust you. Teenage years bring much more danger and require a level of honesty and openness. Otherwise, how can you protect them? If you don't know what they're going through, you cannot possibly protect them.

<u>Superdad Pro-Tips:</u>

1. Don't react to catastrophe. Let the smoke clear so you can think before you swoop in.

2. Let your kids come up with solutions to the next problem in their lives.

3. Remember to just advise. Don't jump in to take control. Let them develop a plan.

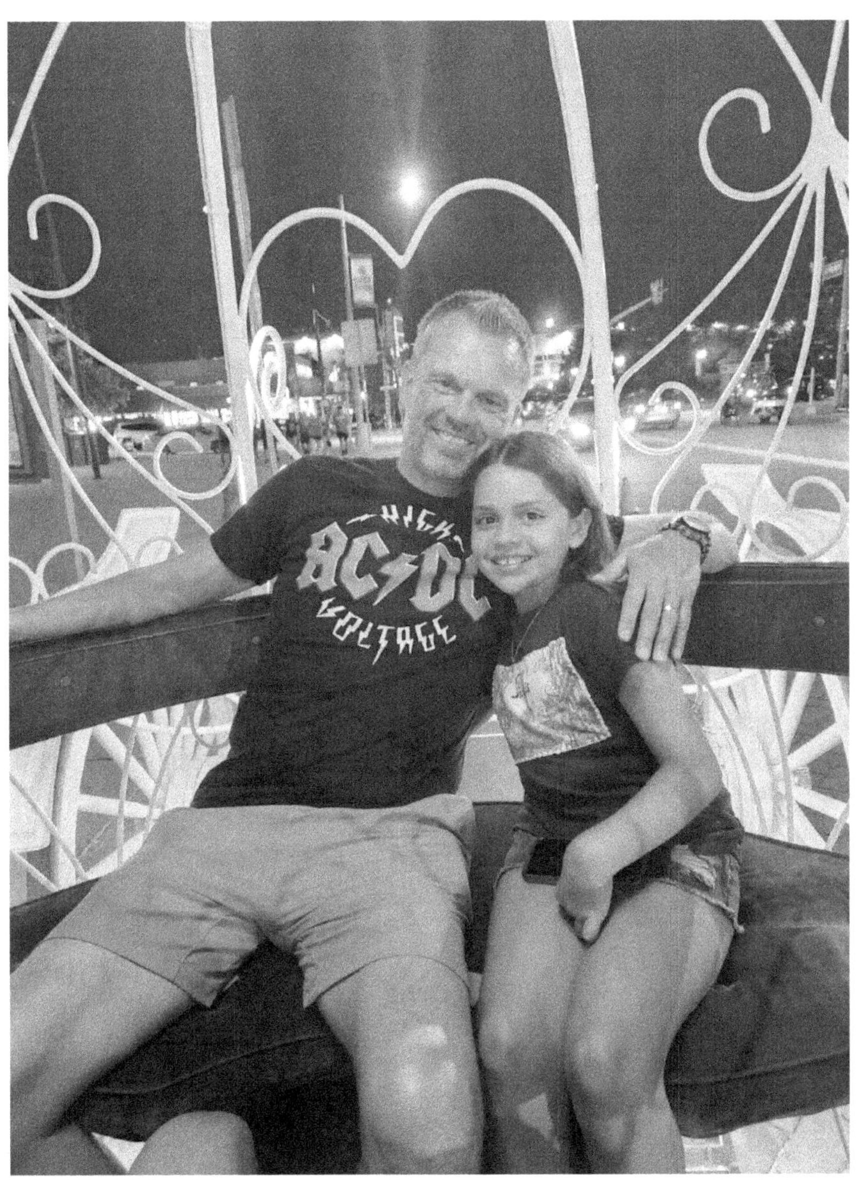

Chapter 7 – Affectionate

"Self-interest is the enemy of all true affection"

-Franklin D. Roosevelt

Talking about affection is really a conversation about your upbringing. What you experience as a child has immense influence in what you believe about affection. It forms how you perceive love. As hard as it may be to look back, this is where we need to do a deep dive and ask tough questions about the patterns we grew up with. Who your parents were and how you were shown love helps you understand the patterns of showing love and affection to your children.

Fran and I grew up in very different environments, yet somehow similar. We both grew up in rough, urban neighborhoods; her in Dallas, and I in Chicago. I grew up with an abusive, sadistic father, drill sergeant stepfather, and hard-working, functional addict mother. Fran grew up with a functional addict father and a hard-working, saint of a mother. We both attended public schools. We both struggled with rules in school. We both only received affection from our addict parent. This would prove to be a real factor in our parenting styles and how we show affection to our children.

Many of us that grew up in abusive environments don't want to admit we are anything like our parents. In fact, most people we meet despise that assertion. I remember once my mother remarked how much I resembled my biological father and it sent me into a rage. She didn't know at the time of all the sexual abuse he inflicted on me. She only knew of the physical abuse. Regardless, my reaction was resent. I hated the thought of looking like someone I hated. Someone who had done so much harm to me and my mother.

I remember saying something similar to Fran one day while we were having a conversation. I pointed out how she hugged just like her mom. Her reaction at first was denial and then grew into silence. I didn't understand at the time that I opened a wound. Between the two of us, Fran is slower to open up. A complete opposite of myself. Doesn't make sense? I know. The abused kid from Chicago is an open book (and writing them) while the girl that never experienced abuse is tight lipped. But I knew at that moment that I hit a nerve and we would have to revisit something important here.

You see, if it really is nothing and it has no power over you, then why react? The mere fact that we are reacting is a universal sign that something is there. We walk through life saying things like, "I'm over them" and "It doesn't really matter, but…" If it doesn't matter, then why is there a 'but?' We lie to ourselves about how much things really affect us. We say these things because we don't want them to bother us. We are in a state of denial about many of the things that impact us, especially our upbringing.

However, when we're talking about our psychology and behavior patterns that impact our parenting, it becomes a much more serious matter. Before we had children, our patterns only affected a few dating relationships and friendships but now our patterns effect our kids. We cannot simply ignore this away because it impacts our children. Now I'm no psychologist or counselor. I know a few and I'm certain they would agree with this statement. If we continue to ignore our parents influence in our ability to parent, we will continue in a very similar pattern. We will be stuck if you will. Stuck in the patterns we experienced as a child because we repeat what we see.

What we learned over the years is that we both resented being compared to certain family members because we didn't want to continue their behavior patterns. My father was cruel. My stepfather was rigid. I had to unlearn almost as much as I had to learn about parenting. Fran's mother was an amazing wife and mom, but rarely showed affection through hugs, kisses, or telling Fran she was loved. We both grew up with deficiencies as it relates to affection and love.

I experienced abuse and rage as a child, so I was predisposed to anger and overreaction. I have struggled with that my entire life. I'm not ashamed to admit it. I ignored the impact abuse on me for years and as a result, I repeated the patterns of overreacting. I've overreacted to everything under the sun. What hurts the most is when I overreacted to my children's mistakes.

When Jayden was young, he played youth sports. I stepped down from my high school coaching job and agreed to coach his team. One game, Jayden exaggerated an injury to imitate my limp, although we didn't know that until much later. I had knee surgery in my twenties that left me with bone on bone in my left knee. The doctor informed me that it would develop into painful arthritis in the future, but as a young man in the prime of his life I did think about the future.

I asked Jayden at every stoppage if he was alright, to which he replied he was fine. I wasn't sure if I should play him. I benched him. He begged to be put back in the game. Jayden limped through an entire game. It was so bad to the point even other parents approached me inquiring about his condition. It was so confounding and embarrassing for me as a parent and coach. I wasn't sure if I did the right thing by playing him.

When we got home from the game, Fran and I asked what was going on? Jayden was a shifty kid, never giving a straight answer. He told us one thing, then another. I wasn't sure what to believe. I overreacted. I started yelling. It was horrible. As silly as it sounds, I overreacted after a youth basketball game because my son was too embarrassed to tell me he was imitating me. How silly is that?

Once we learned what was really going on I had a sit-down with my son. I looked him in his eyes and explained that I was wrong to react that way and that I loved him unconditionally. Jayden accepted my apology and he moved on. What really hurt was the guilt that was now setting in, something I would learn fed my addiction to alcohol. Anger and alcohol are best friends.

In fact, it is for that reason I took so long in writing this book. I have started and stopped for over fifteen years! Every time I would start writing I'd hear this voice, "Who do you think you are? Look at how big of failure you are at parenting. You can't write a book about parenting." Most parents can probably relate to this guilt. We are our own worst critics. We beat ourselves up over our mistakes long after our kids have moved on and enjoying the day.

Anger is my enemy of affection. I have learned over the years that nothing demands an immediate reaction. I don't have to react. I don't have to say anything. Most times it's best for me to marinade and meditate. Get perspective first, then speak or act. We live in such an action – reaction world. It is difficult work and I still sometimes miss the mark, but my mistakes are much shorter lived. As a good friend used to say, "there is no such thing as a bad day, only a bad five minutes."

I've seen enough of my reactions ruining the closeness with my children, and wife for that matter. I finally reached a point that I was willing to shut my stupid pride up and make changes. I faced the reality of my father's influence on my psyche and have worked to mitigate my weaknesses. And that is strength. Real strength.

Fran had a much different enemy of affection. While I was a flash-in-the-pan type of overreactor, I had no trouble showering my children with hugs and affection. My mother and grandmother set a wonderful, loving example of showing affection. Fran was the complete opposite. She had very little affection shown to her as a child. She was the oldest of four children, so her role became more of that of an additional parent. She did not get the hugs and kisses I would receive from the women in my life. Only a maternal grandfather would give her that affection sporadically. Her enemy of affection is coldness.

Fran's mother was brought up in a poor, small town in Mexico. Life was difficult and affection was something her mother did not often show her or her siblings. Chores, duties, and work dominated the day. No time for matters of affection. Fran's mother passed this pattern on to her children, rarely hugging or kissing them during their formative years. I'm happy to say that she has learned that affection is important to a relationship and started giving more affection each time we see each other, especially to the grandbabies.

This is not about who is at fault or some sort of blame game. We must get out the courtroom mindset, where there is a guilty party, and they must be punished. We're working to identify and correct our parenting deficiencies. That is all. Anything beyond this is dysfunctional and going to destroy your progress, and quite frankly is pedantic.

Fran knew she had to address her inability to show and receive affection, but that process would happen on its own time. She needed time to process and accept. That's the thing about change, it happens on its own timeline. We can try to rush it, but it happens organically. It is why I love the song, "You can't rush you're healing," which is playing as I write this, ironically. Yes, another Trevor Hall plug.

How did she overcome being closed off and cold? She faced it and decided that she was going break that pattern for her kids. She commitment to show the kids affection, even if she didn't feel it. They were her motivation. At first, hugs and words of affection were a choice. She set her mind to do it, almost like a discipline. Do you feel like working out or eating healthy every day? But we know those things are good for us. Great, in fact. Eventually the feelings followed. That's the thing about love, it always breaks through, just not in our timeframe.

I'm so proud of Fran's decision to overcome her deficiency to show affection. Most of our marriage, she has watched and supported me to overcome this or that. It is rare that I find myself on the other end. She prioritized our children's mental health and well-being over what felt comfortable. Sometimes we must do things that are deliberately uncomfortable for us, and our children to grow.

Perhaps you weren't shown an example of affection, or you were even abused as a child. We're here writing this for you. There is hope. It takes work. It isn't easy, but our children are worth it. They don't get to choose their parents. We're all they got. Let's show them how to overcome the past. Let's show them affection.

I'm willing, how do I start? So glad you asked! Once you identify your deficiencies and acknowledge change is necessary, I recommend educating yourself on how love and affection is perceived or experienced. We all experience love and affection differently. People from different genders, ages, races, and backgrounds can all have different preferences and receptors as it relates to showing and receiving affection.

I recommend reading the book, "The Five Love Languages" by Gary Chapman. In his book, Gary Chapman lays out five basic patterns in which human beings give and receive love and affection. They are:

1. Acts of service

2. Giving of gifts

3. Quality time

4. Words of affirmation

5. Physical touch

Learning these patterns of communication can help us better express how we feel towards someone, particularly our families. We tend to communicate love in our love language, meaning we give love the way we want to receive it. However, we must learn our family's language to better express love towards them. If my love language is quality time but my wife keeps buying me gifts, it doesn't reach me quite the same as a Netflix and chill would. I appreciate the gifts, but that is her love language.

What is your child's love language? Ask them questions about the five languages. You will need to tailor them to be age appropriate. Physical touch is probably the easiest of the five to spot. You probably already know which of your children is always hugging, touching, etc. Quality time can be harder to spot, especially if there is trauma or walls of resentment.

After finding your kids love language, brainstorm a list of activities, gestures, notes, events, things you can do to show them they are loved. This can be anything. You're just brainstorming. You can always go back and revise of adjust to reflect the weather or seasons of life. Get as many ideas as you can written down in a file. Add to it every time you get a new one. The problem isn't that you can't think of anything to do. The problem is you aren't a good record keeper.

We forget 90% of what we think, and I'm being kind. This is probably higher if you are older or have a history of addiction, like I did. Force yourself to keep notes. You will forget. We're busy juggling work, projects, meetings, grades, practices, games, dentist appointments, bills and we finally get a free moment, and we can't think of one thing *they* want to do. What about leaving it up to them? That depends on the kid. I have one kid that has a choice made in less time than it takes you to read this next sentence, another kid, we could be sitting there for another chapter. Write it down.

Writing down different experiences of love also shows your effort through creativity. You are giving your children a variety of experiences. You're creating their love dictionary. By showing them different examples of love, you're showing them a great example for their adult lives and relationships. I always explain to my kids the beauty of trying new things means it won't always work out. We've done a few things together that we all agreed, we would never do again. But that's the fun of trying something new. You might find your new best thing.

My daughter's primary love language is gift giving. She loves it when Fran and I return from an outing and have something for her. It says to her even though we were out, we thought about her. It can become expensive, but what's a girl Superdad to do? She is worth every penny. She would wrap her belongings and re-gift them to us when she was little, just to see the excited looks in our faces when we opened her gifts. A gift is how to show her love. It doesn't mean the others won't send the message, just not as clear. We look for creative ways to always remember Bella when we're out. Sometimes it's as easy as grabbing a Matcha Latte with extra cold foam. As Sean Connery would say, "An unexpected gift, at an unexpected time, is the key to a woman's heart."

My son, on the other hand, is a bit more complicated. His primary love language is words of affirmation. Sounds easy? Try finding different ways to say, 'I love you' or 'I'm proud of you'. Yep. Not so easy. Jayden is particularly tricky because he is exactly like me. He wants specificity and isn't afraid to seek clarification. For example, just the other day I commented that I was proud of him to which he replied, "for what exactly?" I had to outline his accomplishment of making National Honor Society even with a difficult teacher. I pointed to his commitment to making the Varsity Basketball team. Most of all, I'm proud of his character. He is a good young man, big brother, and son. The most effective use of words with Jayden is not when I'm speaking directly to him. I've found that while I'm talking with a friend or we're at an event, he lights up when he hears me rave about him.

Whatever you find your child's love language to be, search for creative ways to show them love. It's not about how much you know you love them. It's about how well the perceive that love. Perception is reality. It is a totally different conversation than intent. And why not increase your effectiveness by speaking their love language? There is only one of you. Make your efforts exponentially more impactful and watch your children light up!

<u>**Superdad Pro-Tips:**</u>

1. Ask questions that will reveal your child's love language. Record things that wow them.

2. Speak that love language to your child every purposefully each week.

3. Apply this to your marriage as well. It works!

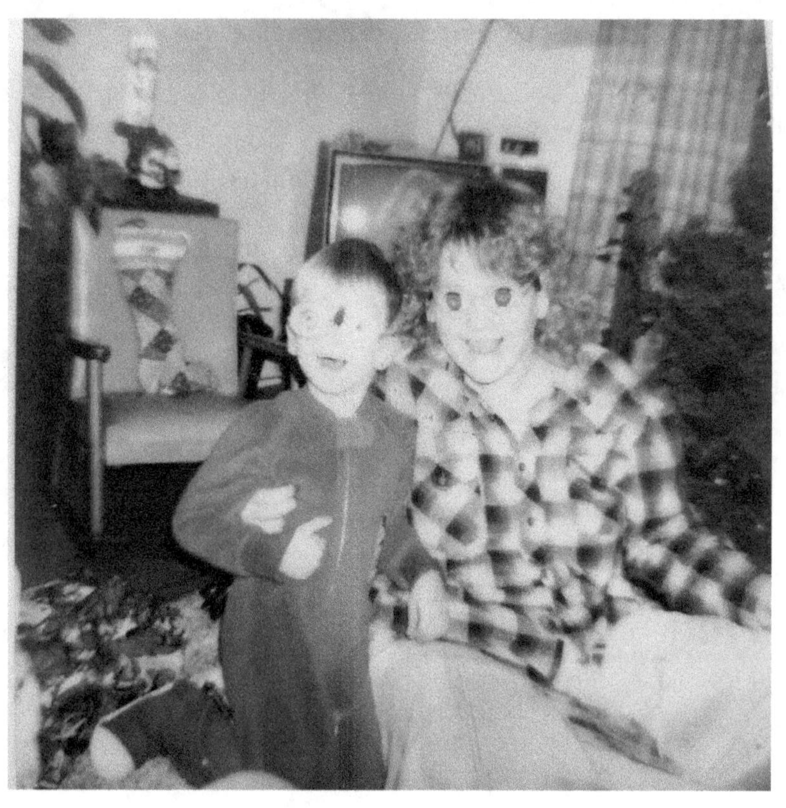

Chapter 8 – Patient

"Don't break the wheel trying to steer the ship"

-Michelle Obama

What wise words from the former First Lady! She raised two daughters during their teenage years in the White House with the entire world watching. Talk about pressure. In her book, Mrs. Obama was asked about this, and her reply helped me understand the trait of patience. We don't have to over-parent. We don't have to react and confront everything at that exact moment. Wow. There it is. Where has this epiphany been for all these years?

This may be the hardest chapter for me to write personally. One compliment I've never received is how patient I am. In our American urban lifestyle patience is no longer a virtue. We're accustomed to immediacy. Patience is more of an annoyance. Whether you're merging onto a highway, standing in line at the grocery store, or on hold for customer service, patience is a lost trait. We are always in a rush. This impatience spills into our parenting and effects our family relationships.

Patience is a sign of intelligence and strategy. Great military generals understand this principle. Focus on the war, not each single battle. Our war, as parents, is raising good kids in a crazy world. As parents, sometimes we get sucked into strife without any forethought. Then we're left with our thoughts of guilt and bewilderment. How did we get to this? We must consistently ask ourselves, is our goal to win the argument or teach our children?

We know once barbs are traded, neither side is listening to the other any longer. Each party is now on the defensive, listening only for a break in the conversation so they may launch their attack. Bad communication patterns are extremely hard to break, especially when each party is separated by decades. Most people only must overcome one bad communication example from their dads. I got two.

As a child I split time between a biological dad that exploded into fits of rage at the drop of a dime and a stepdad that followed the military way. I remember as a small child before my biological parents divorced my father beating up my mother and me. In fact, it is my earliest memory on this Earth.

The argument began at the dinner table. I was too young to understand exactly what the central issue was, but I understood the tone. Voiced were raised. Insults were exchanged. He hit my mom. She attempted to run up the stairs of our apartment. He pursued her upstairs, so I reached out to grab his back jean pocket. I pulled on his back pocket to stop him, he turned around and shoved my down the stairs where I landed.

My father would continue beating my mother until he cracked her head with a house phone as I laid helpless on the floor. A concerned neighbor heard the violence and called the police. My dad avoided arrest because he himself was an officer, and very manipulative. My mother sent me to Las Vegas to live with my grandparents while the divorce was finalized.

Living with such a monster made me afraid all the time. I felt weak. I hated laying on that floor too weak to help my mother who was crying out for help. I developed a friend in anger because it made me feel strong. I didn't realize at the time that I was walking into a bear trap. I would learn the exact same patterns of overreacting in anger as my biological father. This "friend" would hurt my wife and children if left undealt with.

After the divorce, my mother re-married Carter, a friend she met at work. Carter became my stepdad and raised me since the age of four. He is thirty years older than I and communicated through the military filter. Some call it old school. I outrank you so do what I say without question. Listening wasn't his job. It was mine. I would bounce between residences but never had a voice.

He did make sure that I understood the mindset of respect, but not listening. I've passed that respect mindset onto my children, to a degree. I teach my children that every adult should be respected. Whether you are standing in line at lunch, sitting in class, or boarding a school bus, every adult should be respected. Children aren't being taught this enough in my opinion. As an educator, it is the most alarming trend I've seen over the last twenty plus years.

However, I had to learn that the respect mindset should not mean your child has no voice. Communicating with today's teenager is a different conversation. This generation faces more temptations to do wrong than we ever imagined. If you are stubborn and dug in on the concept of old school communication patterns, believe me, you will lose the war. You will helplessly get sucked into arguments. Arguments become unforgiveness, resentment, despair, and isolation.

How do I know, you ask? Because I've made that mistake a thousand times a thousand. I repeated what I was taught by two ineffective and dysfunctional examples: anger and dominance. You are my subordinate. You obey me. Period. If you dare disobey, anger and punishment will teach you not to. I now look back at my younger self with such regret. I cannot express to you dads out there enough, please push the pause button. There is almost never a time when such harshness must be employed.

Instead of creating an employee or adversarial relationship with our children, perhaps we should enact a more strategic approach. Next time you find yourself in a back and forth with your child, don't react. Especially on serious matters of the heart, be very slow to speak. Stop your brain from searching for the next thing to say. Pause the parent mode. Remember how it felt to never have any power. Try and place yourself on the other side. Yes, I know they don't do that. They're children. That's why we must show them how to. There will be time to explain what we are doing and why, but for now let us be the example.

We must constantly remind ourselves of the bigger picture. This requires us to suspend personal pride and the need to be right. Just relax. There is a bigger picture. You can't see it at the moment because anger clouds the mind and ability to think. Ever said something in anger, only to regret it hours or days later? Allow yourself time to restore peace and homeostasis. You don't have to fix it right now. Go for a walk. Listen to music. Pray. Read. I've learned that one strategic conversation with my children is more effective than a hundred shouting matches.

Remember that the words you allow out of your mouth at this moment can and will do damage, potentially for a lifetime. Kids don't remember homework or chores, but they sure do remember our mistakes. To be a

Superdad means you know the point you're trying to convey is important, but you are patient enough to wait for your children to have a lightbulb moment. That moment when a lightbulb goes off in their head and they see exactly what you've been saying for weeks, months, and probably years. At that moment the lesson becomes internalized, and they will have that for the rest of their lives.

Remember that being consistent will only strengthen your point in the privacy of their minds (chapter 3). Most children ultimately know deep inside that their parents are right about what is being said. They just don't want to admit it. They lack the humility to admit they're wrong and need to change. But don't we all need more of that? When is the last time you looked someone in the eyes and admitted to being wrong without a "yeah, but…" or a "what I meant was…"? We humans are so full of diatribes. We judge others by their actions, but we judge ourselves by our intentions.

When you remain patiently calm it tears down the defense mechanisms children employ to discredit your point of view. You can be consistent in your approach because you understand the master plan here. You understand Michelle's words. We don't have to see the result right this second. We will win the war. Our kids will turn out alright because of our persistent patience.

Before you get the wrong idea about my approach, let me be clear. I'm not saying to let everything slide in a feeble attempt to be your child's friend. No way! Children need us to parent, not to impersonate some teenage friend. We talked in chapter 2 about principles. My children know what our non-negotiables are. We have two no-fly zones in our home: respect and truth. They do not change. They are two-way streets. They apply to everyone living in our home.

Not every argument is a serious matter. Many are what I call compound frustrations. Most parents I meet complain about their child's attitude and reaction to tasks. Whether the task is homework, washing the dishes, or taking out the trash, the reaction from their child is generally negative. A roll of the eyes, a sigh, or the "I'll do it later" approach are frequently employed by the American teenager. Many of the parents I talk to describe a frustration with their child's lack of follow through on tasks. And this generally leads to arguments and frustration. Isolation leads to resentment and there you have a recipe for family strife.

Remember we described patience as both intelligent and strategic. Let me ask you a question. Who pays for your child's entertainment? Phone, phone service, internet, Netflix, Xbox, PlayStation, car, insurance, gas, and petty cash probably all comes from you and your spouse. What I'm about to suggest here requires both parents to be on the same page. This will not work if one is circumventing the other to be the more liked "friend," which isn't parenting at all. In fact, we can apply that to most of the strategies in this book and others. Not much will work if parents are not in concert.

Think about your career and what it took to get there. Now think about all the sacrifices you made to provide. We are motivated by compensation. As previously stated in chapter 1 (selfless) our economic system is driven by profit motive. Teens want the profits but aren't motivated. We must be strategic about how to provide the motive. Let's teach our children to work for the extras they want in life. Set agreed upon prices and an accountability checklist for the tasks you want to see accomplished and watch that trash get taken out. We pay our children every Sunday for the tasks they've done.

I can hear some of you asking, "Didn't you say not to have an employee relationship with your children?" Yes, of course we're not talking about employee's when it comes to matters of the heart. In this context, we're talking about mitigating our children's apathy and aversion to work. Let's stop getting upset because things weren't done, or our children have a sense of entitlement and let's do something about it. Stop allowing them to be a mood-altering substance in your life. Let's be strategic about setting up a system of rewards to motivate them.

After all, isn't that what worked and works for us? Profit motive. We stay in the lines and perform well at work because we know we will be compensated. There are different degrees to which I've seen this employed. I had a friend in college who described his parents paying him to work on the family farm. They didn't pay for anything in his life other than essentials: shoes, clothes, and food. If he wanted entertainment, he had to work. This may seem a bit extreme for many of you, and I may agree, but I will admit I've never met anyone with a stronger work ethic on planet Earth than that friend.

We use a simpler approach in our home. We post set prices for jobs and let our children have choice. Do more tasks, check the box, and make more cash. That simple. Fran and I also take on tasks that require daily attention like dishes. She loves to load and run the dishwasher at night. Nothing like going to bed with a clean kitchen is her motto. I love waking early and unloading the dishes before anyone wakes up. This way, there is never an issue with the kitchen and its flow.

Set up a system that works for you and your home. The bottom line is to increase our patience by employing intelligent strategies that reduce stress and strife. Life is stressful enough without petty arguments and getting upset over little things. Save your intense energy for the non-negotiables or principles. Remember our goal is to teach our children lessons, not win an argument. Being right isn't that fulfilling anyway.

<u>Superdad Pro-Tips:</u>

1. Begin with the end in mind. Ask yourself what's really important? Being right or the relationship?

2. Remember that events come and go. Your reactions can last forever.

3. Focus on your humanity and mistakes. You aren't perfect either. When your patience is tested, take five. Take a walk. Breathe. Listen to calming music. Get out of the fire!

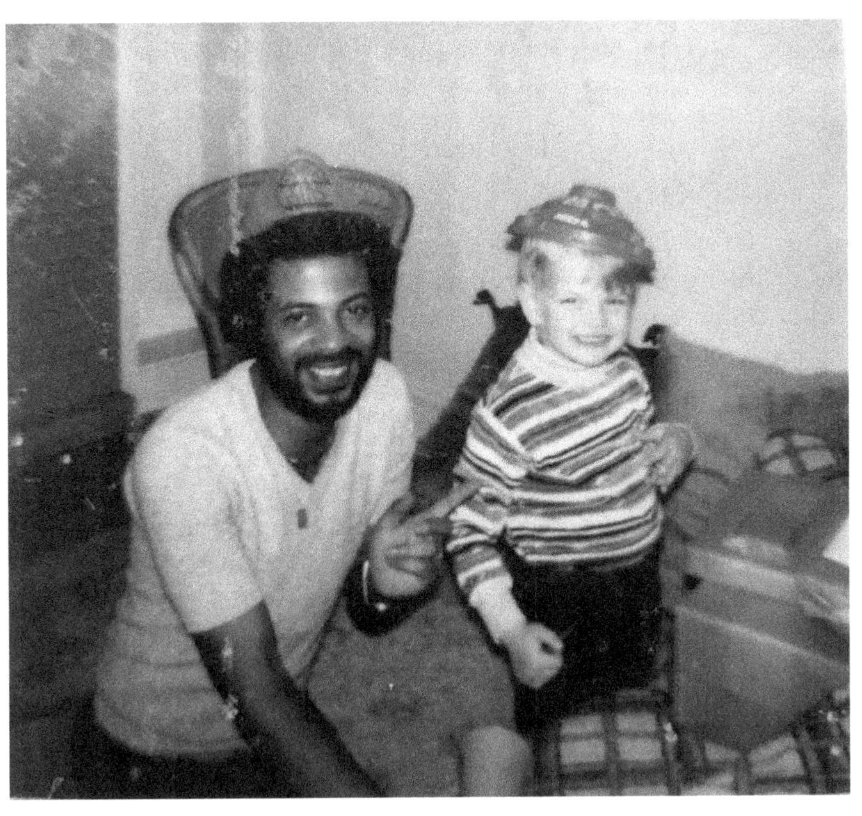

Chapter 9 – Forgiving

"Forgive everything that has ever happened…and let all of your mistakes become all of your greatest gifts in disguise"

-Luka Lesson

Yes, we saved the hardest one for the end. We saved this trait for the end because it really is the heart of the matter. You see, we can embody all other eight traits every single day of our life 150%, but the truth is our children will still fall short and disappoint us. They will hurt our feelings. They will be, well, children. We have two options, hold grudges that erode the foundation of everything we've done up to this point. Or second, we admit the hurt they caused, and decide to forgive.

But we're not only talking about forgiving our children or loved ones here. We're talking about living as an example of forgiveness for your children to follow. A healthy example of conflict resolution that will help them forge healthy relationships and recognize unhealthy ones. This is breaking the cycle of anger and unforgiveness.

True forgiveness means letting it go. Not to bring it back up at thanksgiving dinner trying once again prove we're the right party, only to rip the scab off the wound for it to bleed all over. How many of us repeat the same conversations with our loved ones? We keep doubling down on our point of view as if somehow that will finally bring a different result. They just don't understand, we tell ourselves. No, it's us that don't understand.

We cannot control how others react. What a simple concept, right? We don't get to control how or when someone has an epiphany, apologizes, or stands their ground. We cannot control them, so why do we return to the same arguments repeatedly? Unforgiveness is really about control. Letting go of control means you no longer must prove your case in a court of law. We rest in the truth that we can only control ourselves, our reactions, our words. It is so freeing!

How do I know? I spent most of my life doing the exact opposite. A well-known fact among my family and friends is that I don't stay quiet if something is wrong. Some call it a "clap-back" mentality, while others would've referred to me as "direct" or even "combative". Whatever term we affix, it was a learned behavior that served me well in my childhood as a defense mechanism. Abuse, abandonment, and the streets of the westside of Chicago were all great incubators for this defense mechanism. Always project strength. Always answer back. Or become a weak target and suffer the consequences.

Problem is when I left Chicago and entered college in Dallas, I quickly noticed that others did not behave the same way. As I entered college, I was surrounded by people who were far more mature than I was. They had healthy conflict resolution skills, while I was still fighting and holding onto anger. Was something wrong with me? Why was I powerless to change the way I reacted to situations? It took years of prayer, meditation, and study to pinpoint the exact root of my behavior pattern. I was the problem.

Allow me to save you years of pain, failed relationships, and isolation. Like many of you reading this, I grew up rough. I did not always have great adult mentorship. And the mentorship I did receive was generally in the wrong direction. I looked up to street guys who were tough. No one messed with them and when some poor soul did, it ended badly for the challenger. I admired tough guys because the abuse I suffered made me feel weak and the environment I was raised in glorified toughness. But now I was in college, literally in the safest space of my entire life, and I don't know how to drop my guard. To forgive. To let it go.

If you are like me, you've overreacted so many times the people who are left in your life already know the playbook. Something happens, something is said, you have an instant reaction without any thought for the outcome and anger wins again. Oh, that old friend, anger. He will help you survive in the moment, but then will haunt your relationships and life for the rest of yours. I know the rinse and repeat process all too well, my friend. How many family members and friends watched helplessly? I'm a lucky man they stood by my side and gave me time to heal and change. Thank God they were patient with me.

And what about my kids? My kids didn't ask to be brought into this world. My wife and I made that choice for them. They deserve to have a better example of conflict resolution than blowing up in anger and holding onto unforgiveness. So how do we forgive? There is no easy answer to that question. Just like raising children, there is more than one way. I am sharing what worked for me. This does not imply there is no other path.

I used to believe that if I prayed enough, the feelings of anger or offense would go away. In this sense, anger was a symptom of being carnal, or not spiritual enough. That is so false. Churches and mosques are full of very spiritual people who are holding onto unforgiveness. It's a wonderful perfume, isn't it? Learn the spiritual buzzwords, say the right things, act the right way, and everyone assumes you are fine. We humans are so good at acting.

Real forgiveness starts with self-awareness. We cannot fight what we cannot see. You must see yourself the way the rest of the world sees you but does say anything because they are too afraid of your reaction to tell you. Doing this implies humility. You cannot see yourself as you truly are because like me, you spray the phony perfume of career, education, accomplishments, meetings, and worse, reasoning.

We love reasoning, don't we? Well, did they tell you what they did to me? We reason away our guilt and stay in the bear trap of anger and unforgiveness. What a destructive pattern I was caught in? Reason is the enemy of metacognition and self-awareness because it keeps your mind focused on what they did and not your reaction. Why spend time focusing on what you cannot control?

There is no timetable for self-awareness. It happens organically in periods of sobriety, solitude, and peaceful reflection. You cannot rush self-awareness. But there are things you can do to foster its timing of revelation. I make time every morning to reflect, meditate, listen to music (HUGE TREVOR HALL FAN), write, read, pray, sit by the pool, drink coffee, and get quiet.

This world is so contrary to those things. We allow ourselves to get sucked into this vortex of busyness without any real thought or reflection. We focus on winning favor with the boss, reports, deadlines, projects, sales, and jobs that keep us busy, distracted, and sick. It is an easy trap. Perhaps that is why the world seems to be only getting more and more angry. Driven on a highway lately? Road rage is almost a daily occurrence in Dallas, Texas.

We must make the time. If it is not a priority, we can easily fall back into that vortex and watch years pass by. Real self-awareness will reveal your part in the process. It will show you how others feel. I told you about a difficult period in chapter 3 where my son where he was lying to us constantly. Lies to cover up lies. I was so frustrated. I would yell, punish, spank, and yet nothing seemed to work. He kept lying. It never occurred to me at the time that I was lying to myself about alcohol abuse while chastising him for his lies.

It was a vicious cycle where he would get in trouble, then lie, and I would blow up. This repeated for almost an entire year. During a period of solitude, two things occurred to me. First, yelling and anger isn't working. Second, that this cycle wasn't only affecting my son, wife, and I. You see, my daughter was forgotten in all the anger and yelling. She would run to her room when I would get upset with my son. How sad? I unknowingly created fear in my innocent daughter. How could I be so blind? It is crushing to relive this memory and type these words, but my hope is that it helps you avoid the harm that I caused my family.

Without sobriety and reflection, I would have continued that cycle. I had to change my behavior to break it. I had to make time to get quiet, get sober, and listen. Some days are more fruitful than others. But each day I sit in my backyard and make the time to reflect is a win. Trevor Hall said it best in his song "karma," "Got to break that cycle. Break it strong! This been going on for way too long!"

Now I realize that all this is scary. Telling a grown man who probably overcame great obstacles in their life and made a success of themselves to sit quietly each day may sound crazy. You may be saying to yourself right now, "I don't need to change. They do!" Well, let me ask you, how is that working? Yes, we can point to their blame. My son was guilty. But my message wasn't getting through because I had to break the cycle first. I had to lead by example and be open about the process. Man, that kind of humility is the stuff great relationships are made of!

I'm super pumped to announce that we did see a breakthrough and my relationships with my son and daughter have never been stronger. But it started with me. I had to be willing to change first. You see, holding on to reason will justify your unforgiveness and anger. Unfortunately, it only destroys us and our relationships. Unforgiveness is like swallowing poison and expecting the other person to die from it.

True awareness will always lead to action. Do exactly the opposite of what your brain is telling you when you're angry. Stop reasoning with yourself about why you're mad. Let it go. Put on meditative music and let it carry the anger out of your body. Sounds silly, doesn't it? I know. I laughed too. But it works!

The song "Forgive" by Trevor Hall transformed my life. So much so that I got the word tattooed on my left arm, so I never forget just how important forgiving is. I had such a hard time letting go of people that wronged me. I fixated on what was done to me. As a child, I suffered abuse and neglect of every form. It was easy for me to focus on wrongs. An innate sense of justice, I called it. It was such a destructive thought pattern to model for my children.

As weeks turned into months of sobriety, I quickly started to notice that by focusing on the offense, it only fed anger and unforgiveness. I sat quietly and looked for answers. I questioned myself. Is that how you want to spend your days on this Earth? What if you're living your last days? Would your attitude about being right change if you knew you only had a month to live?

In my first book, "My journey to heal the body" I describe a time where I thought heart disease, high cholesterol and blood pressure may kill me. I will tell you my friend, facing your own futility reminds you what is important. Being right, justified, all seemed so unimportant when I thought I may be living my last days.

My question to you is simple, why wait for a diagnosis to change? Benjamin Franklin said only two things are certain in life, "death and taxes." Life can turn in an instant. One doctor's visit, one blood test, suddenly life as you know it is different. You begin to think about all the missed opportunities to be a better person, husband, father. You recognize in that moment that tomorrow isn't promised and you've wasted a lot of time, assuming it would be.

I'm happy to say that I've made a full recovery, am off all medications, and teaching others about the power of the vegan diet, and more specifically nine superfoods. Whether you're facing a health crisis or not, why wait to embrace what is real until the end? Why wait until you are lying on death's doorstep to connect with you children? Let go of stubborn pride and give it a try. As a dear friend always says, "It doesn't matter who is right. All that should matter is how can we fix it."

We believe that forgiveness is the final trait of a Superdad because offenses in life will come. It is an inevitable truth that relationships + time = conflict. Now, you may read these words and aim to avoid conflict by never getting too close to anyone. I assure you, when the day comes to leave this Earth, you will regret that decision. A Superdad doesn't run from conflict, they accept that it is inevitable and work to fix it.

<u>Superdad Pro-Tips:</u>

1. Predetermine that no matter what happens, you will not hold onto resentment. Remember that holding onto unforgiveness is like swallowing poison but expecting the offender to die from it. It only hurts you.

2. Find a quiet, calming space every day to release stress that spills into your home.

3. Listen to music that calms your storms and encourages you to be a better person.

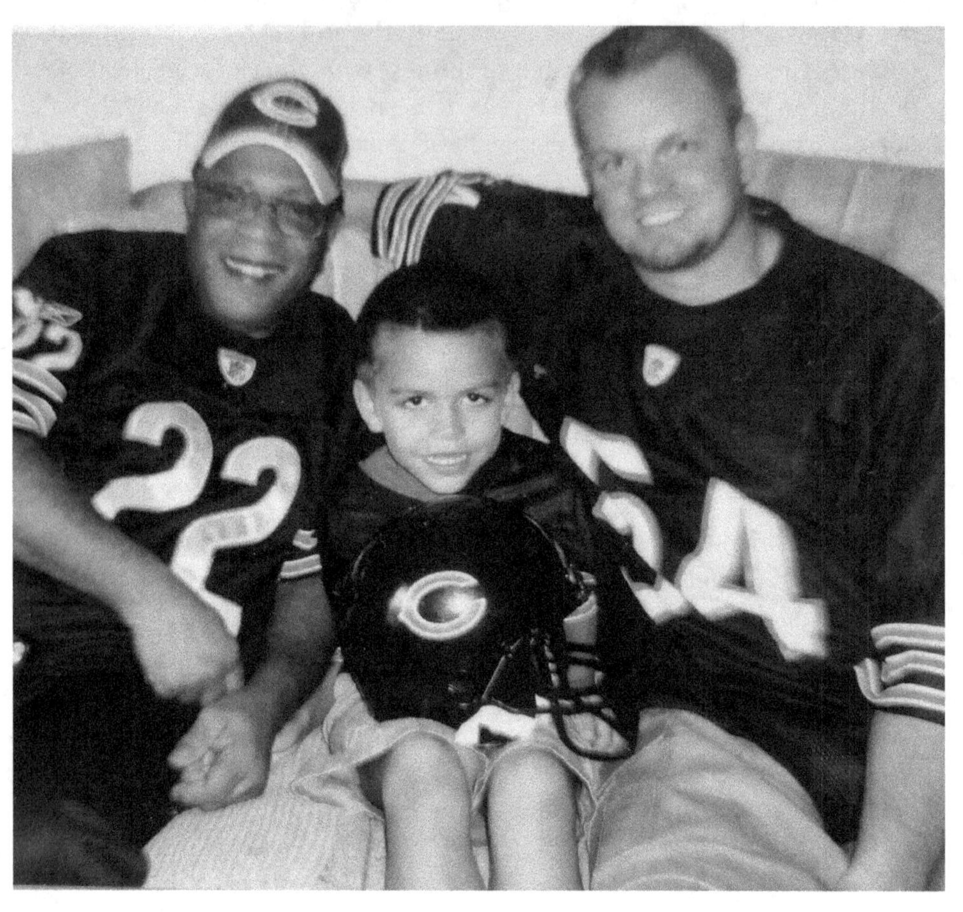

Chapter 10 – Final Thoughts

"It isn't what you do, but how you do it"

-John Madden

Forgiveness doesn't end with your spouse and children. We must forgive ourselves too. Perhaps you keep stumbling in an area and everyone is on your case about it. People remind you of your shortcomings with their quiet look of disappointment. And then you pile on the guilt because no one can torture us like we can. Why do we father's think that is a viable path to enlightenment and change?

Give yourself a gift of forgiveness. So, you screwed up. Get quiet and still. Allow yourself to accept that you cannot change what has already happened. Accept that before you try to do anything else. You cannot erase or rewind what happened. It is over. Leave it there. Now make up your mind to do different, ignoring what your brain and feelings are saying at the present moment.

If you're like me and you are prone to overacting, accept that your family is expecting you to do just that. When you're ready, purposefully walk into the room and change the temperature. Make a joke. Offer to take the family out to eat at their favorite restaurant. Engage your family so they can help reshape your behavior patterns. But make allowance for their doubts too.

Remember this a new for them too. They are conditioned to expect you to overreact, to blow up. We must be patient with their doubts. If we acted in a certain way for years, why would we expect it to be undone in weeks? Above all, keep in mind this is a journey, not a destination. We're changing for the rest of our lives and relationships. This is not a quick fix.

I applaud you Superdads who have dedicated yourself to being a better version of yourself for the benefit of your children. And they may not realize or appreciate that fact until much later in life. We do it because it is what they deserve, not because we seek some award or recognition. We chose to start a family and have children. They had no power in that decision. To that end, we owe them our best. We cannot make up for past mistakes, but we can choose to be a Superdad today.

We may fail over and over, but we keep pushing towards growth. That is what makes us Superdads. Not some phony standard of perfection. No one is perfect. Stop comparing yourself to another parent, dad, or friend and focus on being a better you today. Stop searching for the perfect plan and work on your weakness today. Remember it's not what you do, but how you do it.

I'm always amazed by the different parenting styles. For years I've asked myself 'Am I doing this right?' The insecurity of raising children cannot be matched by any other. You are not matching an outfit or losing weight, you are forming a how a human being will engage in the world for years to come. You are creating standards and principles that will probably last a lifetime. What an honor! We get to mold our kids to help them become better people.

It's not easy. It seems like everything in life is set up for you to fail. As soon as you start working on one trait, you blow it in another area. Been there. Done that. Please don't approach this like I did golfing. I quickly learned how bad I was at my first tournament. I realized how far I had to climb to be good. I didn't want to be that bad for that long just to get good at it, so I quit.

Raising our children is a journey we get to take together. There is no finish line. It isn't a destination. Our kids will eventually catch on that we are not perfect. That's when things get interesting because they no longer look at us as flawless, perfect role models, but see us in our humanity. It is then that they choose to engage in a relationship with us. That is when the real beauty begins. They give us the gift of accepting our faults and loving us anyway. True unconditional love that isn't determined by performance or recency is what all great relationships are built on!

Your children will forget trips you take, vacations you go on, and sporting events. They will never forget how you made them feel. Showing our kids they are valued and loved every day to the best of our capabilities is the path to being a Superdad. This is our journey. We chose this. We accept the things we cannot change right now. We choose to work on the areas we can improve.

Remember that one day you will leave this Earth. You will no longer be there to console, or offer advice, or listen. It is this sobering thought that led me to write this book and four others. You see, I had a medical scare that brought me to a point of recognizing my own futility. It changed the way I saw life, career, marriage, and my children. I wanted to begin moving in a positive direction. I started small. My kids and wife barely noticed. But each day I changed a little more. Regardless of if someone noticing or not, I made moves.

And that is the secret here, making progress each day. I decided that I wanted to be more than an expected role. It wasn't easy. Humbling in fact. But it is so worth it. I always teach my basketball players to not have any regrets. Play the game with all you heart so at the end you can honestly say 'I did everything in my power to help our team'. Approach life in this way. Give your best today. And tomorrow. And the next day. Don't chase some reward or moment. Just do it because it is the right thing to do.

One day you will awake to new relationships that you never thought possible. Until that day, focus on doing the right things. There is no scoreboard, but there is a clock. Our time with our children is so short. Grandparents try to teach this with little success. Most parents are too busy juggling financial responsibilities, family schedules, meals, and work priorities to be bothered with the truth that your days are numbered.

Perhaps that is a harsh reality for some. It was for me. But a sobering one indeed. It led to writing these words and becoming a better man. And that is my prayer for you, Superdad. Don't quit just because you didn't get the reaction you were hoping for. That's weak sauce. Stay in the game. Show your children resiliency by waking up each day and accepting the challenge to work on yourself and become a Superdad.

It may be overwhelming at first, but I promise you it's worth it! Start today. Why wait? Our children are looking for someone genuine, not perfect. We still have time. If we woke up today, we could begin today. I was extremely transparent about my transformation because of the circumstances. You may choose to be more subtle about your efforts That is perfectly alright. It isn't about how start, it's about starting. The longer we sit with this awareness and remain inactive, the less likely change is to occur.

Many adults have learned to move slowly into things. There is wisdom in that approach in most of life's opportunities. This isn't one of them. Our destructive behavior patterns only get stronger with each passing day. Delaying movement, any movement, is feeding the problems that persist. You will figure it out on this journey.

But this journey does not afford any guarantee's this will work. Perhaps in the beginning it gets worse. Maybe your daughter goes off on you the first day. Funny thing about change, it is uncomfortable. Don't be surprised by negative reactions, especially at first. When a child reacts in this way, they're afraid. They are afraid to put trust in you and be hurt. It is a defense mechanism I know all too well.

Be patient. Remember we've allowed destruction in our lives for years and it won't change in hours or days. This is a journey. Keep moving forward with the deep conviction that you are doing right by yourself, your spouse, and children.

Thank you for reading my book. If you need any support on this journey, feel free to reach out at the email address provided in the copyright page.

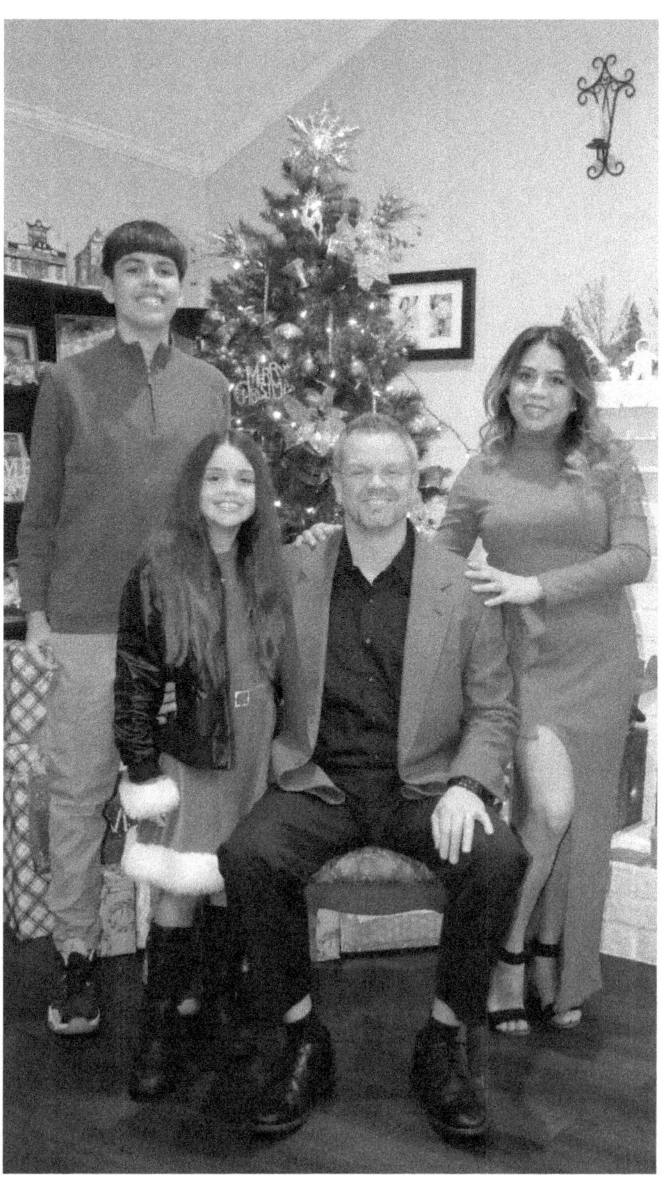